SENSORY PATHWAYS TO HEALING FROM TRAUMA

SENSORY PATHWAYS TO HEALING FROM TRAUMA

Harnessing the Brain's Capacity for Change

Ruth A. Lanius
Sherain Harricharan
Breanne E. Kearney
Benjamin Pandev-Girard

Foreword by Daniel J. Siegel

gp

THE GUILFORD PRESS
New York   London

Copyright © 2025 The Guilford Press
A Division of Guilford Publications, Inc.
www.guilford.com

Printed in the United States of America

This book is printed on acid-free paper.

For product and safety concerns within the EU, please contact
GPSR@taylorandfrancis.com, Taylor & Francis Verlag GmbH,
Kaufingerstraße 24, 80331 München, Germany.

Last digit is print number: 9 8 7 6 5 4

Library of Congress Cataloging-in-Publication Data is available from the publisher.

ISBN 9781462556915 (paper)
ISBN 9781462558209 (cloth)

About the Authors

Ruth A. Lanius, MD, PhD, is Professor of Psychiatry and Harris–Woodman Chair at Western University in London, Ontario, Canada, where she is also director of the clinical research program for posttraumatic stress disorder (PTSD). She has worked with trauma-related disorders as a clinician and researcher since 2000 and established the Traumatic Stress Service at London Health Sciences Center. Dr. Lanius is particularly interested in the firsthand experience of traumatized individuals throughout treatment and how it relates to brain functioning. She has received numerous research and teaching awards, including the Banting Award for Military Health Research, and has published several books and over 200 research articles and book chapters focusing on brain adaptations to psychological trauma and novel adjunct treatments for PTSD. Dr. Lanius regularly lectures on the topic of psychological trauma, both nationally and internationally.

Sherain Harricharan, PhD, completed her doctoral degree in neuroscience at Western University and is currently pursuing a doctoral degree in clinical psychology at McMaster University. Dr. Harricharan's research focuses on PTSD, employing various neuroimaging approaches to study altered neural circuitry patterns among traumatized individuals. Her interests include how sensory processing pathways in the brain are altered as a function of trauma and dissociation, with an emphasis on the influence sensory input can have in shaping higher-order cognitive functioning in trauma, including emotion regulation, social cognition, and attentional processing. Dr. Harricharan has published peer-reviewed articles and presented her work at numerous international conferences.

Breanne E. Kearney, MS, MRes, is an occupational therapist and a doctoral candidate in neuroscience at Western University. Ms. Kearney has over 10 years of experience working in a variety of settings with children and adolescents with sensory processing challenges, using a play- and relationship-based approach. She has received advanced training in sensorimotor-based interventions at the STAR Center in Denver, Colorado. Ms. Kearney's doctoral work in Ruth Lanius's lab involves using neuroimaging to investigate the neurobiology of sensory processing and the efficacy of mind–body treatments in PTSD. She is particularly interested in studying the relationship between sensory processing, attachment, and trauma-related symptoms.

Benjamin Pandev-Girard, MOT, is an occupational therapist in Montréal, Québec, Canada, with a focus on consulting to organizations and supporting individuals affected by complex trauma and dissociation. He is passionate about bridging sensory processing research with practical interventions that meet diverse needs. Since 2021, Mr. Pandev-Girard has collaborated with Ruth Lanius and her trauma research team. He also works as a mentor, clinical supervisor, and consultant for schools, youth protection units, and early childhood centers; offers professional workshops on trauma, sensory processing, and mental health; and is a lecturer at Université de Sherbrooke. Mr. Pandev-Girard is a recipient of the Excellence in Clinical Supervision and Teaching award from the Canadian Association of Occupational Therapists.

Foreword

Ruth Lanius, Sherain Harricharan, Breanne Kearney, and Benjamin Pandev-Girard have created a comprehensive, useful, and fascinating tour of the impact of trauma on the sensory systems of the brain and what we can do to support the journey to healing these deep developmental wounds. Our tour guides offer not only clear, in-depth, and cutting-edge scientific views into the eight senses that shape our experience of being alive, but also practical clinical steps any therapist can harness to catalyze deep and lasting change toward well-being.

Trauma overwhelms our ability to cope. For a young child, these life-changing events can assault the integrity of the body and the sense of relational safety that are fundamental to developing a state of security and a coherent, whole, reliable sense of who we are, our inner "sense of self." The term *self* can be seen to involve three fundamental facets: our *subjective sensation* of being alive, our *perspective* or point of view, and our *agency*—the center of initiating action. This "SPA" of sensation, perspective, and agency form the foundations of self-experience, the here-and-now flow of energy that is the essence of what our "experience of being alive" entails.

When this energy moves in a "bottom-up" direction, we can view this as a raw, direct flow that arises upward into our awareness. We can also experience energy flow that is "top-down," meaning that prior experience molds this flow into a constructed set of representations shaping our direct experience of self—our subjective sensory worlds, our perspectives, and how we have agency, or not, in our lives. Here in *Sensory Pathways to Healing from Trauma* we are given an empowering opportunity to learn how the intricate pathways through which energy flows, in both its bottom-up and top-down directions, are negatively impacted by traumatic experience. As Louis Pasteur said, "Chance favors the prepared mind." This book prepares your mind for whatever interactions arise in psychotherapy and enables you to deeply understand what is going on and how to offer practical guidance toward healing.

Trauma impacts the developing mind and brain by compromising a key process called *integration*. Integration can be defined as the linkage of differentiated elements of a system. Integration is how the self-organization of a *complex* system enables optimal functioning. A collection of elements defines a system, and a complex system is one with three key features: it is *open* to influences from outside of itself, it is capable of being *chaotic*, and it is *nonlinear*, meaning a relatively small input at an initial time can lead to a result that is large and difficult, if not impossible to predict. Complex systems have the process of *emergence*, in which the interactions of the components of the system give rise to something more than simply the components themselves. An example is the wetness of water, an emergent property of the interaction of H_2O molecules that is not present in any single molecule itself.

If we think of our own human lives, we may come to realize how we are immersed in complex systems, and even how we ourselves *are* complex systems. Our nervous system, including its brain, would be one example. But what in fact is the *mind* of our lives? The mind can be said to include four facets: subjective experience, consciousness, information processing, and self-organization. This latter aspect of mind is that emergent facet of complex systems in which they naturally regulate their own unfolding. From this vantage point, the mind can be defined as "an emergent self-organizing, embodied, and relational process that regulates the flow of energy and information." A healthy mind, then, can be proposed to be one that optimizes self-organization. How does this occur? By enabling integration to arise. Complex systems move like a river, bounded on one side by the bank of chaos, the other by the bank of rigidity. The central flow of that river of integration is the result of optimal self-organization that arises when integration—the linkage of differentiated parts of the complex system—is allowed to emerge. When integration is blocked, the system tends to move toward the banks of rigidity or of chaos, or to both. The various symptoms of posttraumatic stress disorder (PTSD) reveal examples of this chaos and rigidity that plague the life of those with unresolved trauma.

Trauma impedes the embodied and relational system of the mind—in both our bodies and in our relationships—from achieving integrative flow. In a given moment of time, this means going beyond the boundaries of what can be called a "window of tolerance," a metaphor for a process that defines a span of activation or arousal that enables optimal flow to emerge. This flow has the FACES features of being flexible, adaptive, coherent, energized, and stable. Across time, those with unresolved trauma will have narrowed windows of tolerance that make their lives prone to moving beyond the window's boundaries and entering states of chaos and rigidity, the hallmarks of unresolved trauma. But beyond this clinical profile of PTSD, a sense of coherence as an inner and a relational self—the SPA—is fractured in these frequent excursions outside the window.

In this powerful and engaging book, you will learn how energy flow through nonlinked networks of the brain has impaired neural integration and altered our eight sensory systems. It is these systems that shape the bottom-up flow of how we come to know the external world and also experience our internal, embodied lives. This blockage of fundamental neural connections can also be seen in areas such as the corpus callosum, the hippocampus, the prefrontal regions, and the interconnections of the connectome (see Martin Teicher and colleagues' foundational research). As bottom-up sensory streams of energy come upward to enter conscious experience, they may be filled with chaos or rigidity. As top-down flow from our higher neural regions tries to make sense of these compromised streams of energy flow that fracture a sense of coherence, further impediments to the integrative making-sense of life block us from living a coherent life of wholeness. Our sensations are restrictive, our constructed perceptions can become hypervigilant for danger, and our agency is repeatedly and exhaustingly focused on defense. In this way, we understandably develop a SPA of a nonintegrated inner and relational self far from the FACES flow of a coherent life.

The brilliant bounty of this book provides a conceptual foundation for every clinician—and coach or parent-educator—to understand the deep impact trauma can have on feeling whole. Taking in these deep immersions slowly and savoring their deep insights is a deeply rewarding journey. By learning about these integrative networks of the brain and how trauma negatively impacts their growth, you as a reader will be ready to take this powerful new information into action. One way to understand this empowering gift is with this adage: "Where attention goes, neural firing flows and neural connection grows." In the Bridging to Practice sections of each chapter you'll find practical tools for directing your client's attention in ways that will promote the growth of neural integration in networks whose differentiation and linkage has been compromised by trauma. These clinical interventions will harness the power of attentional focus to direct the neuroplasticity that activates new neural communication for your client. Attention is the superpower you will learn to harness for yourself as a clinician and for your clients in their pathway to healing and health. With this new attentional focus, neural firing is activated, which can turn on the genes to produce the proteins needed to grow the new synaptic connections, sometimes new neurons (in the hippocampus especially), and even lay down the myelin sheaths—all in a developmental therapeutic process that will enhance neural network connectivity. In other words, your guided attention can stimulate the growth of new differentiation and linkage in your client's brain, promoting the growth of neural integration at the heart of well-being. With the exciting new conceptual knowledge and focused clinical interventions awaiting you in the pages ahead, you will be prepared to promote the neural integration that will help your clients widen their windows of tolerance, resolve their traumatic histories, and live a life of meaning, connection, coherence, and wholeness.

DANIEL J. SIEGEL, MD
Clinical Professor of Psychiatry, UCLA School of Medicine,
and Executive Director, Mindsight Institute

Preface

The idea for this book has emerged over the last two decades, during which we have had the privilege not only to observe the resilience and perseverance of traumatized individuals but also to bear witness to the stories of their suffering and their healing journeys. In serving as honored witnesses, we have come to see how the brain adapts to trauma.

Through the brave trauma survivors who have participated in our research, we have gained a wealth of knowledge into the effect trauma has on the brain, mind, and body. As one individual once told us after we looked at her brain scan together, "I now know that it is my *brain*—it is not me." This statement inspired us and shaped our purpose for writing this book. Our aim is not only to help translate what we have learned about the brain to clinicians, showing how the brain in the aftermath of trauma drives the perception of the world and how we react to it, but also to provide clinicians with insights to use with their clients aimed toward the restoration of the self in the aftermath of trauma.

This book focuses on how trauma alters how sensory information is processed in the brain, thereby affecting individuals' perception of themselves in the world. There are eight sensory systems processed in the brain: vision, hearing, taste, smell, touch, vestibular, proprioception, and interoception. We describe how traumatic experiences can be viewed as insults to the body's eight sensory systems and how this directly shapes how individuals perceive both the internal world of their body and their external surroundings.

The book is divided into nine chapters, each focusing on a unique aspect of sensory experience in the aftermath of trauma. We recommend that you read the chapters in order, since each provides knowledge with a "Bridging to Practice" feature that offers brain-guided healing tools that can be applied to clinical practice. We have also provided cases in each chapter, drawing on our own experiences and those of contributors.

Chapter 1 describes the neuroanatomy of sensory experience and its relevance to trauma. It also provides some foundational knowledge about neuroplasticity and how it can facilitate healing from trauma. The "Bridging to Practice" feature provides tools for a sensory inventory of a client's experience following trauma.

Chapter 2 provides an overview of how sensations are processed, identifying key regions in the brain critical to processing different types of sensations. We also introduce how some of these structures work together to form networks that guide our attention when encountering these sensations. The "Bridging to Practice" feature offers guidance as to how individuals can become more attuned to safe sensations within their environment.

Chapter 3 highlights how sensory experience is processed differently when one feels safe or unsafe. Critically, we discuss how feeling unsafe largely limits sensory experience to the lower preconscious level of the brain, causing an individual to react without thinking. The "Bridging to Practice" feature provides exercises that help individuals identify safe sensations that maximize the engagement of the cortex, therefore allowing them to experience a fuller range of human potential and providing the foundation for cognitive interventions.

Chapter 4 describes how sensory experience can inform the nervous system's line of defense. When these innate lines of defense are activated, the lower brain becomes the "decision maker" and orients to sensations from the threat in order to mount defensive responses that maximize chances of survival for the traumatized individual. The "Bridging to Practice" feature provides clinical insights into how to manage different types of defensive responses and how to avoid pitfalls that can frequently be encountered in a clinical setting.

Chapter 5 shows how the sensory experience of balance is critical in shaping how safe an individual feels in the world. A sense of safety provides a springboard to freely experience the sensory environment, fostering curiosity, agency, and play. The experience of balance maps onto the brain's vestibular system, which includes a dense network of connections involved with processing both the external world and the internal world of the body. The impact of trauma on the balance system and its brain networks is described. The "Bridging to Practice" feature provides exercises aimed at reclaiming one's center of gravity after trauma.

Chapter 6 introduces the sensory system of interoception and discusses how visceral sensations are experienced in the brain, mind, and body after trauma. The brain pathway for interoceptive sensations converges at the level of the insula, where individuals become aware of these interoceptive sensations that contribute to the feeling of being alive. This contrasts sharply with frequent descriptions of feeling emotionally numb and dead inside from traumatized individuals. The "Bridging to Practice" feature provides clinical insights that can support an individual through the process of identifying shifting visceral sensations and understanding how this inner emotional turmoil is connected to their feelings of unsafety. Reinhabiting the body in this way fosters the feeling of being alive with one's self and others.

Chapter 7 illustrates how the world is perceived through the eight senses and how they are all integrated to provide a unified perspective of the external environment. The translation of sensory information to key brain networks involved in the perception of the external world can be profoundly affected by trauma. Clinical insights in the "Bridging to Practice" feature help to link sensory experience with the window of tolerance discussed in Chapter 4, as a means to help facilitate embodiment and shift perspective of the world toward a felt sense of safety.

Chapter 8 focuses on how an altered sensory perception of the internal body and the external environment can lead to a fragmented sense of self after trauma. After trauma, the sense of self may sometimes only be perceived as somewhat intact and alive when there is extreme sensory input involving hyperarousal, threat, and terror. Here, we discuss how brain networks dealing with trauma-related sensory experiences involving arousal and raw negative affect can become coupled with the brain network underlying the sense of self, creating a trauma-related identity. The "Bridging to Practice" feature provides clinical insights aimed at helping individuals feel whole and alive in the present.

Although the brain has adapted to trauma, **Chapter 9** describes how its innate malleability can lead to healing. This chapter explores how the integration of top-down and bottom-up therapeutic approaches can be tailored to each individual to restore the self and enable the individual to foster meaningful social bonds with others and build a sense of community. The "Bridging to Practice" feature provides clinical insights that support self-reflection on the part of the therapist, which in turn empowers traumatized individuals to harness their natural capacity to heal.

We hope that this book aids in making the invisible wounds of trauma visible, thereby reducing the shame and stigma that are so frequently experienced by trauma survivors. Our goal is to teach clinicians about the imprints of sensory insults on the brain and provide clinical insights aimed at restoring the self in the aftermath of trauma. Overall, we hope that this book furthers the study and application of personalized, neuroscientifically guided interventions that harness the neuroplasticity of the traumatized brain and support healing.

Acknowledgments

Writing this book on sensory pathways to healing has been a deeply rewarding journey—one that has ignited our passion and expanded our understanding in ways we never expected. Over the past 2 years, every meeting, every conversation, has been a chance to grow together, exchanging insights, challenging each other's perspectives, and building a richer, more comprehensive approach to healing. The process has been more than just a wonderful collaboration across different generations of trauma clinicians and researchers; it has been a shared experience of learning, evolving, and uncovering new depths of knowledge.

First and foremost, we would like to express our deepest gratitude to the survivors of trauma who have courageously shared their stories and allowed their experiences to guide our work. Your resilience and strength are the foundation upon which this book was built.

We are also immensely grateful to our countless colleagues and mentors in the field of trauma, whose wisdom, guidance, and unwavering commitment to healing have profoundly influenced our understanding of trauma and its treatment. Thank you for your thoughtful feedback and ongoing encouragement, and for challenging us to think critically and compassionately about the work we do.

A special thank you to the therapists and practitioners who shared their real-world experiences and therapeutic insights. Your practical knowledge has been invaluable in making this book as relevant and accessible as possible.

We would also like to acknowledge our family and friends for their endless support, patience, and belief in us throughout this process. Your understanding has kept us grounded and motivated.

Lastly, to the countless individuals whose lives have been touched by trauma and healing—your resilience continues to inspire us every day. It is for you that this work exists, with the hope of contributing to the healing and transformation that you so richly deserve.

Thank you all for being part of this journey.

Contents

Introduction to the Senses
and the Sections of the Brain

Nature has placed mankind under the governance
of two sovereign masters, pain and pleasure. It is
for them alone to point out what we ought to do
as well as to determine what we shall do.
—JEREMY BENTHAM (1780)

To say that the brain is a complex organ would be a massive understatement; the human brain is one of life's greatest mysteries. Nevertheless, our understanding of its intricate inner workings has deepened exponentially in an era of modern neuroscience, necessitating ongoing efforts in bridging this knowledge to clinical practice. Thus, this book is meant to help translate what we have learned about the brain to clinicians working with the sometimes confusing, oftentimes debilitating symptoms related to psychological trauma. This knowledge is not only power, it is validation for both clinicians and those with lived experience who can begin to see trauma-related symptoms not as defects but instead as brilliant brain-based adaptations for survival. In particular, this book aims to show how the brain drives our perception of the world and in turn our behavior, and how this is altered in the aftermath of trauma. It also informs treatment approaches that address the whole brain—including the parts inaccessible to language or cognition—and thus promotes transformational restoration through the brain's innate capacity to rewire.

This first chapter provides an overview of the three main sections of the brain: the reptilian brain (the survival brain), the limbic brain (the emotional learning brain), and the cortical brain (the reflective brain). As a whole, the brain's utmost purpose is to make sense of our internal and external experiences through gathering, processing, and interpreting information from our senses, and then direct how we respond. Importantly, these processes involve each section of the brain to varying degrees. Our physical, emotional, and cognitive worlds arise from these three layers, and they are continuously shifting in the context of the felt stability and safety of the body and its surroundings. The shock and horror of traumatic experiences throw an individual's internal and external worlds off-kilter and act as insults to the body's eight sensory systems, directly altering internal and external perception. These eight sensory systems include touch, proprioception, vestibular (balance), vision, hearing, taste, smell, and interoception.

This chapter provides a foundational understanding of how the brain flexibly adapts to trauma as sensory information is detected, processed, filtered, integrated, and translated through each section. We also discuss how sensory engagement is initiated during the attachment relationship and can therefore be profoundly affected by early life adversity. Furthermore, it addresses how recalibrating sensory processing and integration in the brain and body opens the gateway to healing and neuroplasticity, or the brain's natural ability to change and heal itself, after trauma. This provides hope for pathways that can lead to the restoration of brain functionality, which is critical for alleviating the suffering of traumatized individuals. Neuroscientifically guided treatments that can regulate and restore brain networks are highlighted given their potential for helping traumatized individuals feel safe, connected, and belonging to themselves and to the world.

Trauma: An Insult to the Eight Sensory Systems

Traumatic experiences can be viewed as sensory insults, which have a profound effect on how sensory information travels through the brain. The body has eight sensory systems, each of which is described briefly below.

Touch: The Boundary between Self and Other

Our skin is the largest organ of the body, which amounts to the size and weight of a bowling ball when amalgamated (Linden, 2016). It serves as the main physical barrier between our body and the outer environment. The functions of touch are multifaceted, from distinguishing between pleasurable and painful stimuli for the purposes of survival to discovering the world inside and around us. Modestly and discretely, touch helps to form the basis of human connection by promoting a felt sense of safety and attraction toward an attachment figure even before birth. Our body consists of a map of touch receptors that are differently distributed across various regions, with the densest concentration on the highly sensitive palms of our hands and soles of our feet. There are different types of touch receptors located in various layers of the skin, making it very rare for them to be stimulated in isolation. There are also different types of pathways depending on the type of information the receptor detects—for instance, slow pathways (C-afferent) carry pain, temperature, and light-stroking touch information, while fast pathways (A-beta) carry discriminative touch information needed to localize touch in order to effectively navigate our external world.

For example, if you spill a cup of hot coffee on your hand, the fast pathway helps you to quickly detect the cup's perturbed orientation and move it upright to avoid further spilling—however, the burning pain experienced on your hand is registered a couple seconds afterward via the slow pathway. In another example, if one is stroked by a loved one's gentle touch, communication between slower moving fibers creates a feeling of being soothed, protected, and cared for, which underpins the essence of being human (Kearney & Lanius, 2022; McGlone, Wessberg, & Olausson, 2014; Olausson, Wessberg, Morrison, McGlone, & Vallbo, 2010).

From the lens of trauma, physical violence and interpersonal trauma are dehumanizing experiences where touch can be used to threaten and harm. Touch can be used therapeutically in that the exploration of safe touch sensations can help the brain relearn that touch is not always dangerous and can be used to foster safe connection with others and the world at large (see Plate 3.1).

Proprioception: Anchoring the Body in Space

Humans and other animals have the ability to complete movements without visual input based on having an intrinsic spatial map of the body in relation to its environment. This spatial body map is created and maintained through sensory feedback from the body's muscles, joints, and skin stretch receptors, collectively known as proprioception. For example, imagine having dinner during a power outage and your surroundings go pitch-black. Our proprioceptive sense allows us to know where to reach for our cutlery, as guided by the intrinsic spatial map in our mind. It also helps us to complete actions with the least amount of effort since it allows us to know where our body is in space and what amount of force the task requires. In this example, we remain seated at the dinner table while reaching for the cutlery rather than standing up and contracting additional muscles in our legs because our intrinsic spatial maps know where the cutlery is in relation to the body. We recruit only a small amount of muscle fibers to pick up the cutlery; alternatively, when we pick up a glass that we expected to be empty but instead is full of water, we automatically recruit more of our musculature to compensate and avoid spilling the water.

Overall, proprioception guides movements of limbs through space using balanced muscle contraction, with a minimal amount of effort, thereby allowing energy to be conserved (Johnson, Babis, Soultanis, & Soucacos, 2008). Receptors involved in proprioception lie deep within our muscles and joints and are activated through tensing our muscles and stretching tendons or skin, such as when walking or embracing others. Each new experience helps to reinforce the intrinsic proprioceptive map, allowing it to be continually updated in order to anchor the body in space.

When we feel threatened, muscle groups are subconsciously primed for action, or fight-or-flight (Crenna & Frigo, 1991), or inaction, like freeze/tonic immobility or shutdown (see Chapter 4 for more information). When these muscle groups are repeatedly activated under a sustained state of threat, the focus shifts toward an avolitional defensive action instead of engaging in planned, balanced, and precise movements (Kozlowska, Walker, McLean, & Carrive, 2015; Lanius et al., 2017; Mobbs et al., 2007; Schauer & Elbert, 2010). These muscles become chronically activated, causing muscle stiffness, which requires a surplus of energy to comply with the body's demands (Lakie & Robson, 1988). Continual feedback from tense muscles can also influence the areas of the brainstem where proprioceptive input is first integrated, having a cascading effect on brain functioning. Furthermore, various stress and sex-related hormones can have a profound effect on proprioception, causing bodily awareness to fluctuate, from the clumsy peri-pubescent adolescent who bumps into everything to the overworked executive who drops their phone multiple times per day.

During and after trauma, proprioceptive maps can be altered and body awareness (and thus its functionality) may be severely impacted when encountering traumatic reminders, fueling an experience of feeling unsafe and utterly ineffective or helpless. Through movement in a safe environment, proprioception can be transformed from automatic defensive action to more planned, balanced, and precise movements. Ultimately, this can translate to a greater sense of agency and control over one's body.

The Vestibular System: Moving with Purpose

The vestibular system is a consistently activated yet mainly subconscious system working tirelessly to maintain our balance, muscle tone, and center of gravity. Although we are often unaware of its subtle workings, it is impossible to ignore when it is highly stimulated, such as when we accelerate on a roller coaster, or when it is not functioning properly, such as during episodes of vertigo or bouts of car sickness. Head movements activate tiny hairs and crystals within the vestibular sensory organs of the semicircular canals and otoliths, respectively, which are located in the inner ear. These receptors detect the downward pull of gravity and help maintain our body's center of gravity, allowing us to feel grounded and connected to the Earth. Vestibular input plays a major role in integrating and modulating information from other senses, such as proprioception, vision, touch, and auditory systems, in order to maintain balance, coordination, and rhythmic movement (Ferrè, Vagnoni, & Haggard, 2013; Goldberg et al., 2012). The vestibular system allows us to develop adaptive postural reactions when walking on an uneven surface or when otherwise encountering a threat to our physical safety, engaging the appropriate extensor muscles, and positioning our head and neck to analyze our surroundings. Since it orients us during traumatic experiences, it may need to be involved in reorienting the brain and body to safety during the healing process.

Interestingly, it also engages areas of the brain related to arousal and awareness of inner visceral sensations that guide emotions (Harricharan, McKinnon, & Lanius, 2021; Harricharan et al., 2017; Lopez, Halje, & Blanke, 2008); this is easy to consider when we feel acutely aware of the excitement (or fear) and the dropping sensation in our gut during an amusement park ride.

As extreme alterations in arousal and negative alterations in cognitions and mood are part of the core symptomatology of posttraumatic stress disorder (PTSD) and other trauma-related conditions, the vestibular system plays a key role in the compromise, and also the restoration, of physical and emotional balance: feeling safe again in the body and the environment. By therapeutically incorporating and facilitating movement, we can exploit the power of the vestibular system to restore balance and foster a sense of safety, thus promoting connection, curiosity, and joyful discovery of the world. This sensory system is explored in depth in Chapter 5.

Vision: More Than Meets the Eye

The visual system reflects the world around us and continuously receives messages from the environment that are transformed into a visual scene in the brain's vision hubs in the midbrain and occipital cortex. Visual signals create a link between the motor and emotional systems in preparation for action (Anastasopoulos, Naushahi, Sklavos, & Bronstein, 2015). Following trauma, the visual system often becomes hypervigilant to visual cues associated with the original trauma, leading individuals to perceive even innocuous details in their environment as a threat (Kleim, Ehring, & Ehlers, 2012; Lanius et al., 2017). The constant attention to visually triggering cues can be exhausting and energy depleting, also causing the individual to lose perspective and lose touch with the joys of everyday life. Conversely, trauma can also lead to hypovigilance of visual cues, where an individual may not register blatant visual details, such as the face of an assailant from a traumatic memory, or may recall memories only in black and white, thereby facilitating detachment from one's surroundings (Janet & Prince, 1907; Lebois, Seligowski, Wolff, Hill, & Ressler, 2019). Treatment can be directed toward orienting to the present, where individuals can be encouraged to focus on safe visual stimuli in their surroundings, such as certain colors or images in a room that have a grounding effect. This can provide a visual anchor that can help them reorient from being triggered toward finding safety in the present.

Hearing: Your Emotional Sonar

Hearing involves binding together the location and intensity of sound. The auditory system has evolved to filter background noise to support focus on relevant sounds and other stimuli or tasks. It is also trained to recognize the emotion in someone's voice without relying on the other senses (Adolphs, 2002). However, the ability to filter background noise is limited during times of stress or threat, as we become hypersensitive to sounds that may increase or decrease our chances of survival or finding safety (Javanbakht, Liberzon, Amirsadri, Gjini, & Boutros, 2011). This hypersensitivity to sound can cause us to feel fixated on sounds and exaggerate the acoustic startle response, which can disrupt the concentration required for day-to-day tasks (Siegelaar et al., 2006). After trauma, the ability to calm down after such startles is compromised, further disrupting our daily functioning. Alternatively, clinical experience has shown that hyporesponsiveness to sound can also occur after trauma, where individuals are detached from the sounds around them. Treatments directed toward reappraising sounds through safe experiences, such as through music at various frequencies, can help facilitate a new steady state of the nervous system (Porges & Rossetti, 2018; Rodwin et al., 2023).

Gustatory System: To Each Their Own Taste

Have you ever experienced nausea following the consumption of a certain food? Even though the nausea may not be due to this food, chances are that you will be aversive to it the next time you eat it due to the powerful connection between taste and memory (Eskine, Kacinik, & Prinz, 2011). The gustatory system detects five core tastes—sweet, salty, sour, bitter, and umami—in addition to responding to an array of physical features, including temperature and texture. The gustatory system maintains reciprocal interactions with the other sensory systems. For example, taste is influenced by not only the sight and smell of food but also the sounds heard while eating. Interestingly, the gustatory system is also embedded in our common language—for example, one can describe a traumatic event as leaving a "bad taste in the mouth," or a feeling of disgust (Chapman, Kim, Susskind, & Anderson, 2009). Disgust triggers adaptive behaviors aimed at removing or destroying the agent that caused this feeling.

To date, little research has studied the consequences of psychological trauma on taste—however, a limited ability to detect disgust has been shown in response to lesioned brain areas associated with taste (Calder, Keane, Manes, Antoun, & Young, 2000; Moll et al., 2005). Furthermore, loss of taste has been shown to cause psychological distress, as observed following viral infections, such as COVID-19 (Dudine et al., 2021). Importantly, the pleasurable sensations arising from taste, specifically sweetness, are a critical part of forming social bonds with others and feeling connected to the world at large (Schaefer, Kuhnel, Schweitzer, Rumpel, & Gartner, 2023).

Olfaction: Smelling Is Remembering

Often referred to as the oldest sense, olfaction is the sense of smell that evokes affective (emotional) responses and adaptive reactions. For example, scents of environmental hazards, such as fires or predators, elicit fear and terror, whereas scents from decaying material or rotten food elicit disgust. Although odor molecules are invisible to the naked eye, scents are pervasive throughout the environment. When taking a whiff of something rotten, odor molecules activate hair cells in the nose cavity, which are then directly relayed to the olfactory center of the brain (Croy, Drechsler, Hamilton, Hummel, & Olausson, 2016). However, you may habituate to a scent, whether pleasant or unpleasant, if it is deemed nonthreatening.

Scents are processed in memory centers of the brain to give contextual reminders of familiarity from other experiences with a specific scent. If the smell of alcohol or cologne was detected on an assailant's breath during an assault, the victim may become quickly distressed by the benign smell of alcohol or cologne in the environment. Since our sense of smell is intimately connected to emotional experience, disruption of smell can lead to a profound decrease in quality of life. Following trauma, faint scents that were associated with terror during traumatic events can become overpowering and all consuming, flashing the individual back to the time of the original trauma (Daniels & Vermetten, 2016; Pellegrino, Farruggia, Small, & Veldhuizen, 2021; Vermetten & Bremner, 2003). However, olfaction may also be a powerful ally through a newfound felt sense of safety when trauma-related negative emotions are uncoupled from triggering scents.

Interoception: The Gateway to Feeling Alive

Interoception refers to the visceral sensations arising within the body that inform and impact physiological homeostasis, or the body's steady state, as well as emotional processing. Detection and integration of internal sensations with other sensations orient us to the most salient inner cues given a situational context. This allows our body to inform us of danger or comfort and subsequently seek out resources or situations that enable us to operate at our full potential. As an adaptive example, we may feel a visceral fluttering in anticipation of a big exam, which motivates the behavior of studying. Visceral sensations, including body temperature; hunger or satiety; thirst; nausea; and other abdominally arising sensations, such as fluttering or emptiness, inform the imprints of positive and negative emotions, which are the pillars of our intuitions, our sense of vitality, and the depth of our connections with others. For example, a loved one's touch can generate feelings of warmth and a visceral calmness, which foster emotions like love and compassion. Inner bodily sensations converge at the level of the brainstem, which initiates reflexive adaptive reactions to the environment. These sensations can also reach the higher emotional centers of the brain, which operate at a conscious level (Harricharan et al., 2021). Here, we can consciously appraise these raw, visceral sensations and identify the emotional labels associated with them, allowing us to act with intention and meaningfully connect with those around us.

Following trauma, the circuits of interoception are disrupted, which manifests in a range of experiences, including mistrusting the body's feelings, emotional numbness, avoidance of previously threatening or unsafe visceral or physiological sensations, and even an extreme feeling of being emotionally dead inside (Kaye

& Krystal, 2020; Schulz, Schultchen, & Vögele, 2020). This can make it difficult to feel love and connection with the self and others, even those closest to us, profoundly severing communication between the brain, mind, and body. Regaining tolerance and trust in one's bodily sensations is an essential part of becoming whole and feeling alive after trauma. Finding solace through the brain, mind, and body connection can help reclaim interoceptive safety and allow us to fully inhabit our body, opening our hearts to connection after trauma.

The Three Interconnected Sections of the Brain

The brain is our ultimate control center, constantly receiving messages from our surroundings and from within the body. It weighs only about 3 pounds but has been estimated to consist of almost 100 billion brain cells, called neurons, that are in constant communication with one another in order to make the brain function (Herculano-Houzel, 2009; Hubel & Wiesel, 1979). The brain is connected to the rest of the body through the spinal cord, with the two structures together forming the human central nervous system. All animals have nervous systems, including reptiles and mammals, which serve as the main processing hub of the body (Crick, 1979; Hubel & Wiesel, 1979). However, the human brain is the most highly evolved because it allows us to volitionally control our behaviors, think, and reflect on our emotions, as well as utilize long-term memories and language (Bassett & Gazzaniga, 2011; Dehay & Kennedy, 2020; Nauta & Feirtag, 1979).

The brain's direct connection to the spinal cord provides a gateway for connection to the rest of the human body. Through this connection, the brain coordinates the release of hormones to the body and receives feedback from bodily sensations that correspond to our emotional state (De Kloet, 2004; Derryberry & Tucker, 1992; Makino, Hashimoto, & Gold, 2002). However, while the functions of the brain are universal across humans, they are also unique to each person. No one's brain is the same, which is why behavior varies from person to person. Each brain has unique constellations of neuronal communication that are constantly adapting and changing. The patterns of the brain can be shifted by each new experience, further shaping our behaviors and how we feel (Sapolsky, 2015). This is why memories are important for learning—however, their effects can also be felt within the body. This can be a blessing and a curse. As we describe throughout the book, traumatic memories can evoke bodily sensations linked to emotional experience, which can strongly influence brain patterns and shape maladaptive behavior. However, by teaching the brain and body to manage these sensations and emotions, the brain's patterns can adapt and make new connections that help restore balance.

While the brain is a complex organ, it can be considered as having three sections, which have been referred to as the reptilian brain, the limbic brain, and the cortical brain according to the triune brain theory developed by Paul MacLean

(1990). In his theory, MacLean postulated that these brain sections operated independently—however, we know from vast neuroscientific literature that all sections of the brain are tightly interconnected and work in tandem with one another to facilitate all human functions (see, e.g., Janacsek et al., 2022). While MacLean's original triune brain theory may be an oversimplification of this intricate organ, it provides a useful framework that incorporates all levels of the brain, where lower levels of the brain have been largely ignored in modern cognitive neuroscience literature (Janacsek et al., 2022). For example, our brainstem is positioned lowest and closest to the body to help it respond quickly and instinctively for survival-oriented functioning, such as modulating respiration, heart rate, arousal (wakefulness and sensory attentiveness), and blood pressure. Critically, these functions are commonly disrupted in the aftermath of trauma, necessitating a model that considers the brain in its entirety, including the brainstem. For the purpose of this book, we refer to the brain in three sections: the survival brain, the emotional learning brain, and the reflective brain. While these three brain sections are in constant communication with one another, they are each delegated a few specific functions as described below (see Plate 1.1).

The Survival Brain

The survival brain (Plate 1.1, red) is the base section of the brain and is largely made up of the brainstem and midbrain, making it the gateway that connects the brain to the rest of our body through the spinal cord. As we see later, the brainstem is hardwired to maintain physiological functioning via the autonomic nervous system (ANS). The structures in the brainstem that are of particular significance for our later discussions include the superior colliculus, the periaqueductal gray, the locus coeruleus, the parabrachial nucleus, the reticular activating system (RAS), the cerebellum, and the vestibular nuclei, as well as the vagus nerve and associated structures where the vagus nerve enters and exits the brain (solitary nucleus, dorsal motor nucleus of the vagus, and the nucleus ambiguus; see Plate 1.2 for location of each structure).

The main goal of the survival brain is to *survive*—therefore, every reaction it coordinates is in the interest of immediate safety. Our most raw and visceral emotions originate here. The survival brain is also responsible for relaying incoming sensory information that is perceived around us and within the body to the upper sections of the brain. Its function is similar across animals and humans. In other words, it is highly evolutionarily conserved, and for good reason: All animals must prioritize survival and reproduction to conserve and propagate the species. The survival brain can see, hear, and feel at a very basic level outside of our conscious awareness. Most of the sensory information that we perceive around us and within the body enters the brain here. For example, when you have a gut feeling, your survival brain is first to initiate a response. The survival brain coordinates instinctual responses, where we subconsciously react without thinking. This is often initiated during a traumatic event since the reflective brain would react too slowly. When the survival brain reacts, it usually happens quickly and suddenly, which can lead to impulsive behaviors.

The Emotional Learning Brain

The middle section of the brain is responsible for emotional learning, sometimes called the limbic brain (Plate 1.1, blue). In this book, we highlight the thalamus, the hypothalamus, the amygdala, the hippocampus, the striatum, and the ventral tegmental area (see Plate 1.3 for location of each structure). It is often hidden when looking at pictures of the brain because the structures are located mainly in the inner or midline parts of the brain. The limbic brain is a key intermediate between the survival brain and the higher cortical reflective brain, translating key incoming sensory information from the survival brain to shape perspective and emotion processing in the cortical brain. The brain regions in this section are responsible for emotional learning, storing past memories, and controlling the release of hormones (Rolls, 2019).

The emotional learning brain receives sensory information that enters the survival brain and integrates it with content from past memories (Catani, Dell'acqua, & Thiebaut de Schotten, 2013; LeDoux, 2003). Raw emotion(s) linked with sensory information coming from the survival brain arrives at the amygdala, which influences emotional learning (Fosha, 2005; Panksepp & Biven, 2012). The amygdala can influence the strength of emotion attached to incoming sensory information (LeDoux, 2003). Not only does it influence emotion in the context of the current environment but it is also involved in shaping the emotional perspective of past experiences. If the amygdala attaches strong emotion like fear or terror to a particular memory, a single reminder of it can train the emotional learning brain to respond with fear when faced with future similar sensations or situations (Milad et al., 2009; Richter-Levin & Akirav, 2000).

The Reflective Brain

The top section of the brain is the cortical brain (Plate 1.1, green), which can be referred to as the reflective brain. The structures in the reflective brain that we largely focus on in this book include the various domains of the prefrontal cortex, the insula, the anterior, mid and posterior cingulate cortices, the precuneus, the temporoparietal junction (TPJ), the superior parietal lobule, and the pre- and postcentral gyri (see Plates 1.4a and 1.4b for the location of each structure). The cortical brain allows for many advanced functions, including critical thinking, planning, and reflection on past experiences to help understand their meaning and control our emotions. It communicates with the lower brain sections to receive and modulate incoming sensory information. The reflective brain can integrate multiple sources of sensory input at the same time to develop a behavioral response, and it also aids in emotion processing to help inform our perspective on an experience (Wallace & Stein, 2007).

Behavioral responses to our surroundings in the cortical brain are vastly different from those of the survival brain, where individuals subconsciously react without thinking. The cortical brain consciously plans behavioral responses after reflecting on one's thoughts or intentions, one's bodily state, and the sensory information presented in an individual's surroundings (Kayser & Logothetis, 2007; Maier, Chandrasekaran, & Ghazanfar, 2008). There are also areas of the reflective brain that do not primarily take in sensory information but instead store past information or plan for the future. Here, the reflective brain can bring context to a sensory and emotional disposition and modulate one's response accordingly. The ability to develop measured behavioral responses to our surroundings is most optimal when an individual feels calm, grounded, and safe. The reflective brain is also essential for emotion regulation, which is a primary target of rehabilitation after trauma. This helps to control emotional reactivity and related arousal in order for people to feel more connected to their surroundings (Golkar et al., 2012; Kropf, Syan, Minuzzi, & Frey, 2019). Finally, the reflective brain monitors how we perceive ourselves and mediates the social bonds we feel with others.

The Interconnected Brain

In summary, the three brain sections are tightly interconnected and rely on one another to function. For example, imagine the survival brain as the foundation of a house, the emotional learning brain as the frame of this house, and the reflection brain as its roof. If something goes wrong with one part of the house, it can have a domino effect on the others because they are so interconnected. Therefore, rather than focusing on one area of the brain, it is imperative to think of the brain as a whole, with an emphasis on the relationship *between* each of the three sections.

Early Development, Attachment, and Sensory Maps

Babies are born with instinctive drives and abilities that allow them to discover people and objects in their surroundings. Discoveries of the external sensory world and the visceral sensations that our surroundings evoke within us first occur with scaffolding from our relationship with our caregiver(s) and are a key part of early development. Children start to develop connections with the outside world and to their own bodies and begin to reflect on these incoming sensations around age 2. From here, the capacity to envision mental states in self and others starts to emerge, as explained through theory of mind (Flavell & Miller, 1998; Frith & Frith, 2005).

Beginning in infancy, humans develop sensory maps, which are areas of the brain that respond to sensory stimulation and are modulated depending on context, awareness, and past experience (Berardi, Pizzorusso, & Maffei, 2000). Since the discovery of the sensory world occurs at such an early age when infants are reliant on parental involvement for survival, it is natural that the attachment relationship between children and their caregivers serves as a critical determinant for the perception and processing of incoming sensations from the body and its surroundings (see Kerley, Meredith, & Harnett, 2023). Sensory integration theory (Ayres, 1972; Lane et al., 2019) describes how an individual senses, registers, and interprets information from the environment to elicit an *adaptive* behavioral response, one that is situationally relevant, successful, and measured in intensity. *Sensory modulation* is defined as the ability to regulate and organize sensory input and respond in a manner that is graded relative to the nature and intensity of the sensory information at hand (Brown, Tse, & Fortune, 2019; Dunn, 1997).

In secure attachment relationships (Bretherton, 1992; Kerley et al., 2023; Lyons-Ruth & Block, 1996; Schore & Schore, 2008), the caregiver matches and modulates the nature and intensity of the child's affective experience. This attuned experience engenders interpersonal synchrony between child and caregiver, which fosters exploration and natural curiosity in the child. By contrast, an insecure attachment relationship involves an inconsistency in affect between caregiver and child, where being "out of sync" is likely to make a child feel more vulnerable, unsafe, and alienated from others and their environment.

Disrupted attachment can predispose individuals to hypervigilance, an extreme state of alertness, stemming from the young child's desire for protection (Farina, Liotti & Imperatori, 2019; Lyons-Ruth, 2003; Schore & Schore, 2008). Furthermore, a disrupted attachment relationship (Lyons-Ruth, 2007) can also cause the child to be more withdrawn from their surroundings, stemming from a learned helplessness to engage the caregiver. This can be observed in cases of neglect or, alternatively, repeated and inescapable abuse, where fighting back is futile and poses a further threat to safety. Feeling withdrawn from an individual's surroundings can lead to sensory deficits and blunted arousal, where one disconnects from inner visceral sensations and sensations from the external world (Cohn, 2021; Engel-Yeger, Palgy-Levin, & Lev-Wiesel, 2013; Harricharan et al., 2021; Kearney & Lanius, 2022; Kerley et al., 2023; Levit-Binnun, Szepsenwol, Stern-Ellran, & Engel-Yeger, 2014). Insecure attachment in early childhood may then impact adult relationships, which often serve to re-create the affective dynamics experienced with primary caregiver(s). An abused child enters abusive relationships, a neglected child entertains emotionally distant partners. The attachment cycle is one that continues.

In summary, sensory maps in the brain are representations of the internal and external world that guide our feelings, behaviors, and thoughts. Sensory maps are created throughout our development, first in the context of our primary caregivers, and ultimately determine how the brain, mind, and body synchronize to facilitate a dynamic equilibrium of "in-sync" frequencies. However, brain frequencies that are not in unison or that are "out of sync" with the body can be a critical factor underlying the brain–body disconnect that is often observed in the aftermath of trauma (Kearney & Lanius, 2022; Thome et al., 2022). As such, targeting feelings of safety and connection to the body and its concomitant internal and external sensory experience is a key component of transformational, whole-brain interventions for trauma, which hinge on a process called neuroplasticity.

What Is Neuroplasticity?

Neuroplasticity refers to the natural ability of the brain to change, adapt, or heal itself. The brain has an incredible ability not only to change but also to adapt structure and function in response to diverse sensory experiences. It was originally thought that neuroplasticity was limited to short, critical periods during early development—however, research has shown that the capacity for the brain to adapt continues throughout the lifespan (for review, see McEwen, 2013; Shaffer, 2016; Voss, Thomas, Cisneros-Franco, & de Villers-Sidani, 2017). This offers tremendous hope since it implies that the brain has the capacity to recover from physical and psychological injury.

Neuroplasticity can be facilitated and regulated by several factors critical to brain functioning, including neurotransmitters, hormones, growth factors, the extracellular environment surrounding neurons, myelin (insulating sheath that surrounds neurons), dendrites, glial cell activity, properties of membrane and ion channels, genetic predispositions, and experience (for review, see Voss et al., 2017). Sensory experiences, including social connection and mirroring, emotional experiences, exercise, learning new tasks, meditation, and psychotherapy, as well as stress and traumatic experiences, can all be highly influential on the brain (Fisher, 2017; Siegel, 2010). The quality and quantity of sensory experiences play an important role in the nurture versus nature debate, where healthy brain development and the development of sensory maps representative of one's internal and external worlds depend on exposure during critical periods where the brain is optimally malleable to sensory inputs. Nurturance from caregivers is essential to binding these sensory inputs into reliable maps while also creating lasting connections that shape one's future experience with felt human connection.

This brings us to the good and the bad of neuroplasticity. Enriched sensory environments (for review, see Voss et al., 2017), where the caregiver is attuned to and mirrors the child, can facilitate neuroplasticity by optimizing the growth of new brain connections that promote the development of cognitive and emotional systems integral to mental and physical well-being. By contrast, impoverished environments (for review, see Voss et al., 2017), as observed during the psychological and/or physical absence of an attachment figure, can also influence neuroplasticity processes, thereby negatively impacting brain development (Teicher, Samson, Anderson, & Ohashi, 2016). An adverse childhood environment forces the brain to adapt to chronic inescapable threat at the cost of being able to fully integrate all sensations foundational to human experience, including those responsible for purposeful action, meaning making, social bonding, and feeling part of the world at the cortical level (Nakazawa, 2015; Yehuda, Halligan, & Grossman, 2001). Scars from childhood trauma can leave the individual feeling alienated from themselves and the world around them, trapped in a state of terror where the past is ever present and the future is hopeless.

Fortunately, the capacity for the brain to change and adapt throughout the lifespan has been increasingly documented. Studies have shown brain changes in both nontraumatized and traumatized populations in response to various interventions. In nontraumatized populations, exercise, cognitive training, mindfulness meditation, yoga, and exposure to classical music have all been shown to lead to neuroplasticity changes and enhanced cognitive and/or emotional functioning (Cassilhas, Tufik, & de Mello, 2016; Davidson & McEwen, 2012; Hötting, Schickert, Kaiser, Röder, & Schmidt-Kassow, 2016; Santaella et al., 2019). In traumatized populations, studies are also increasingly pointing toward positive neuroplasticity changes in response to a variety of treatments, including cognitive therapy, mindfulness interventions, neurofeedback, and medication, thus underlining the possibility that the brain and body can rewire to recover from traumatic stress (King et al., 2016; Lanius, Frewen, Tursich, Jetly, & McKinnon, 2015; Nicholson et al., 2020; Santarnecchi et al., 2019; Siegel, 2010; for review, see Malejko, Abler, Plener, & Straub, 2017).

This book focuses on how neuroplasticity can be harnessed to facilitate healing from traumatic stress through safe sensory experiences that facilitate engagement and optimal integration across all sections of the brain. We also argue that positive, safe social environments provide the foundation through which neuroplasticity can be facilitated. Interestingly, findings show that holding the hand of one's spouse as compared to holding a stranger's hand and being alone can decrease the brain's response to a threatening stimulus in regions involved in processing emotions and threat (Coan, Schaefer, & Davidson, 2006). Feeling safe and connected to others can therefore be a powerful method for calibrating the brain, mind, and body connection.

Interweaving Bottom-Up with Top-Down Interventions

Top-down therapies for trauma are primarily cognitive therapies—they rely on higher-order cortical functions to challenge negative thoughts and beliefs as a means of facilitating emotion regulation. However, if primitive sensory insults from the initial trauma(s) are not addressed through bottom-up therapies (see below), the cortex may be suboptimally engaged (Harricharan et al., 2020; Lanius et al., 2010; Nicholson et al., 2017; Yehuda et al., 2015), which may render cognitive treatments less effective. Transformational change must occur at the root.

To mitigate this potential barrier, we propose that safe, sensorimotor-based or informed approaches can facilitate a dynamic equilibrium between top-down and bottom-up regulation of the brain, mind, and body, thus optimizing healing practices. Here, we suggest that sensations and arousal at the level of the survival brain, which, in turn, drive our thoughts at the cortical brain level, lead to the notion "I *sense*, therefore I am" rather than "I think, therefore I am." The latter view has led to the long-standing fallacy that the mind and body are two separate entities as postulated by René Descartes. Research is now demonstrating that brain, mind, and body are tightly intertwined and inform one another through a dynamic interplay between bottom-up and top-down neural processes. Targeting physiological regulation through bottom-up processes takes a whole-brain approach by addressing, not neglecting, lower levels of the brain. This can lead to profound reverberations on self-perspective at the level of the cortical brain, which influences how we see ourselves and the world. This is particularly relevant for individuals who do not respond to top-down treatments and are deemed treatment "resistant" or "unresponsive." These damaging misnomers label the individual as defective, instead of identifying the treatment needing to be optimized.

Throughout the next chapters, we illustrate how to harness the natural ability of the brain to heal and restore the sense of self and other in the aftermath of trauma. Recalibrating sensory maps through bottom-up and top-down processes is posited to correspond with shifts in brain activation, connectivity, and frequency patterns. Experientially, this manifests as safer and more bearable internal and external worlds. This can empower the traumatized individual to reinhabit their body and establish a sense of belonging and interconnection, forging a path to leave their unsafe and forsaken world behind. Consequently, the individual enlivens and reclaims inborn capacities for purposeful action, emotion regulation, connection, synchrony, and fulfillment (see Bridging to Practice 1 for additional guidance about how to implement in a therapeutic setting).

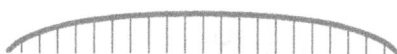

BRIDGING TO PRACTICE 1

Taking a Sensory History: Understanding the Relationship between Trauma-Related Sensations and Arousal

When traumatized individuals are discussing past traumatic experiences, therapists often ask "How do you feel?" This question targets the reflective brain and asks individuals to make meaning of their experience at a time when it may not be fully realized. Instead, we propose taking a sensory history of a traumatized individual's experience by observing and asking about the sensations they experienced during this time. This is critical since traumatic events are frequently not accessible through language and are instead relived as fragmented sensations and dysregulated arousal. A complete inventory of all sensations involved in trauma can provide a framework for a deeper understanding and processing of the individual's experience and response to trauma. This allows the therapist to meet the client at their sensory experience because they frequently cannot express the depth of these sensations in words. This should be done at a pace that feels safe to the client. The therapist should reflect on this as the client is telling their traumatic experience, asking clarifying questions when needed. We have outlined a guide that a therapist could use during their initial session with a client.

Sensory Inventory of Traumatic Experience: An Example

Event (brief description):
A car was T-boned by a truck and spun several times. The client was driving the car and turned their head to their spouse in the passenger seat. Their spouse was frozen and appeared dead. After a few minutes, the client saw their spouse breathing and realized they had lost consciousness.

External Sensations	
Tactile	• Neck pain • Hands gripping the wheel • Bracing of their shoulder against the car seat • Foot on the brake pedal • Wincing of the face You can also ask the client about temperature, pressure, and texture. You can also have the client map out the sensations using the diagrams below. 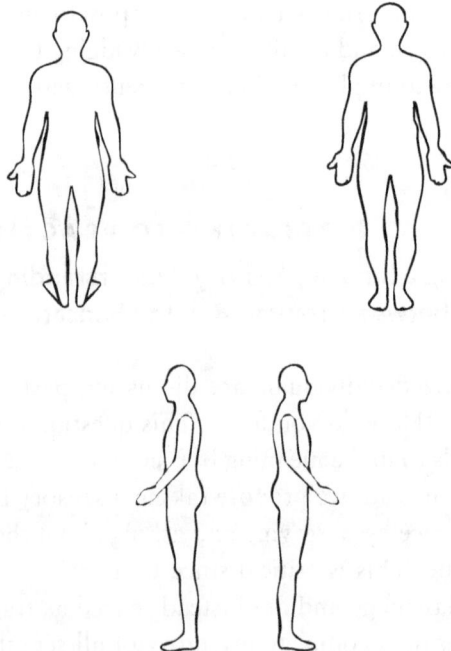

Auditory	• Screeching of the tires • Crash sound of the collision • Scream of the spouse You can also ask the client about tone, prosody, and location relevant to sounds.
Visual	• Sight of husband looking dead • Seeing the airbag suddenly inflate • Dusky skies due to sunset at time of crash • Flashing car lights in the periphery You can also map the client's visual field as they describe the traumatic event (e.g., distance, gaze orientation, location of objects in their environment). Visual Field Distance
Olfactory	• Smell of burning rubber from the tires • Smoky smell from airbag Ask about what words they might use to describe the smell.

Gustatory (taste)	• Dryness in the mouth • Dust in the mouth Ask about the type of taste (e.g., food, alcohol, drugs, genital fluid).

Internal Sensations

Vestibular	• Position of head during trauma:
	  ○ Sat upright in seat and experienced whiplash
	  ○ Head turned toward their spouse
	• Direction of movement:
	  ○ Linear acceleration from whiplash
	  ○ Rotational acceleration from the T-bone impact and looking over to their spouse
	Ask about active or passive head movements made during the traumatic experience. *Note:* Passive head movements (e.g., the car being hit) can often elicit more arousal than active head movements.

Proprioception	• Tension from gripping the steering wheel • Tension from bracing their shoulders during accident • Neck tension from whiplash • Tension associated with shock response upon seeing spouse Ask about active (e.g., gripping, walking) or passive (e.g., impact from being hit) movements made during the traumatic experience.
Interoception	• Hands feeling cold • Nausea from looking at their spouse • Heart racing • Shortness of breath • Chest tightness • Pit feeling in the stomach For the sensations above, you can ask the client to rate the strength of these sensations from 1 to 10.

2

A Sensational Journey

HOW SENSORY INFORMATION
TRAVELS THROUGH THE BRAIN

We do not see things as they are,
we see things as we are.
—ANAÏS NIN (1961)

The senses are the gateway to our experiences, but it is the brain that interprets these signals, weaving them into the fabric of our reality. We are constantly receiving sensory information from the world around us and from within the body. We receive sensory information from the outside, including sight, sound, smell, taste, touch, and vestibular information about our body's current relationship with the downward pull of gravity. Sensory information can also arise from within the body, including our sense of our own body map (proprioception) and interoception: pain, temperature, hunger/thirst, and changes in arousal. Both avenues for incoming sensory information converge at the survival brain.

Typically, the survival brain translates incoming sensory information to the upper sections of the brain to form a perspective of our surroundings and respond accordingly. However, if the body feels threatened, the survival brain can initiate an instinctive coordinated response. Specifically, two intimately connected structures in the brainstem, the superior colliculus and the periaqueductal gray, are critical for receiving and integrating information related to threat or high emotional significance and work in tandem (Steuwe et al., 2014). The superior colliculus is where sensory information about our surroundings enters the brain, whereas the periaqueductal gray receives information stemming from internal bodily sensations and touch (for review, see Terpou, Harricharan, et al., 2019). These two regions are also responsible for swift defensive responses without recruitment of the emotional or reflective brain sections, saving precious time needed to thwart a threat.

Basic raw emotions also emerge at the survival brain—namely, the periaqueductal gray. Neuroscientist Jaak Panksepp (2004, 2005) described seven primal emotional brain systems that originate in the periaqueductal gray of the survival brain, including the FEAR, RAGE, CARE, SEEKING, LUST, PANIC, and PLAY systems. Panksepp deliberately capitalized the words when naming these systems to differentiate them from their colloquial usage and because they are so fundamental to our beings, existing across multiple animal species from reptiles to humans. We theorize that these raw emotions link with incoming sensory information from the body and the superior colliculus to influence how and what information is relayed to the limbic and cortical brain sections. Below we provide two case examples to illustrate how lower-level sensory and raw emotional information processing is altered in the aftermath of trauma.

The Case of Jeremy: War Comes Home

Jeremy is a 48-year-old veteran who was deployed to Afghanistan on several occasions. Jeremy was a member of the infantry, where he was regularly engaged in frontline conflict. During his deployments to Afghanistan, Jeremy's life was repeatedly threatened by the Taliban. He also witnessed three of his close friends being blown up by land mines, and he lost two of his comrades to suicide. Even though Jeremy continued to function throughout his time in the military, his life took a significant turn for the worse after he was released and began transitioning to civilian life.

Jeremy felt that he lost his sense of purpose and structure in his daily routines once he returned, making the transition home particularly challenging. He felt increasingly lost in the world and began experiencing severe reliving flashbacks, where the terrifying events he had experienced in Afghanistan felt ever present. In addition, Jeremy became more and more hypervigilant and no longer felt safe anywhere. He was constantly scanning his environment, and was startled by any noise or sensation that remotely reminded him of his time in Afghanistan. For example, Jeremy felt on edge every time he was playing with his children because he would become preoccupied with background sensations ranging from hearing rustling leaves to seeing strangers pass by. In anticipation of threat, he was distracted by these sensations because they were coupled with remembrances of precipitated rocket attacks. One of Jeremy's most significant triggers was hearing fireworks, since they most closely resembled the rocket attacks he experienced in Afghanistan. Because he felt as though he could be attacked at any time, his inner turmoil reflected his view of the world as a terrifying place. Jeremy therefore became increasingly obsessed with protecting himself and his family from harm. He installed cameras in every room and in every corner of the house. He also began carrying an exacto knife at all times and found that he could only sleep with a gun under his pillow.

Jeremy's family was devastated by how profoundly he had changed after his military deployments. Both his wife and two children were frightened by him as he became increasingly rigid and unpredictable due to his excessive preoccupation with threat. His wife kept begging Jeremy to seek help. However, he was very reluctant due to his inherent mistrust of others, and it took several years for him to finally reach out for support. Jeremy was fortunate to meet a therapist who had a deep understanding of military trauma and mind–body treatments. His therapist also understood the importance of not just helping Jeremy but also involving his family in his treatment. Jeremy's symptoms of hypervigilance and paranoia gradually decreased over time. As this occurred, Jeremy's wife and children started feeling safer at home, and his children were able to function much better at school due to feeling less burdened by their father's inner turmoil. In family therapy, they could safely discuss the implications of Jeremy's difficulties in all aspects of their lives and make sense of their origin.

The Case of Shane: Where Home Becomes a Battlefield

Shane lived in a suburban home and had a typical life until he was 14 years old. He was supported by a loving family that found ways to help him thrive. When he was 3 years old, Shane had a terrifying experience when he had tubes inserted in his ears. He was involuntarily held down by the medical staff without his parents present in order to be given anesthesia. Unrelatedly, at the age of 5, Shane was diagnosed with Tourette's syndrome, a neurodevelopmental disorder characterized by motor tics. Because of his early medical trauma, he was always scared of any medical setting or procedure, which complicated his treatment for Tourette's syndrome. Despite these fears, Shane maintained a lively personality and thirst for exploring the world around him.

When he entered high school, Shane experienced heightened school-related stress and subsequently started to develop more visible tics. When attending his regular follow-up at the local hospital, Shane and his family were encouraged to seek the "best" available treatment at the time: restraint therapy. His parents were hesitant at first, but with the promise of a decrease in tics, Shane told his parents he wished to go ahead with this therapy. This treatment consisted of six sessions lasting 1 hour each, where his hands were tied to a hospital bed by a behavioral support worker, and he was simply instructed to "control [his] tics." Shane felt powerless and deeply ashamed when receiving the treatment because he was unable to control his tics, and he felt like he failed. Sadly, it was through this process that Shane and his family's life changed forever.

After completion of the therapy, Shane continued to develop new tics at an alarming rate. For example, he developed scream-like vocalizations, and his arms would lift up in a defensive posture, leading him to hit his forehead. These tics were severe enough to cause bruising on his forehead and dislocation of both shoulders. This led to havoc for Shane and his family, and their lives became consumed by the severe tics. The tics led to multiple hospitalizations, including surgery to correct the dislocation of his shoulders. The hospitalizations took a toll on Shane's tics since they reminded him of both his childhood medical trauma and of his failures during restraint therapy. The intensified stress from the hospitalizations exacerbated his tics, creating a vicious cycle. His parents felt utterly helpless during Shane's paralyzing distress, to the point where they lost the strength to visit him in the hospital.

Shane's explorer spirit was crushed as he became fearful of every sensation in his body and environment. His parents' neutral gaze and soothing voice were perceived as aggressive and judgmental, and their proximity and touch were experienced as a looming threat. Every outside sensation felt like a potential land mine for a tic explosion. Shane eventually became confined to his living room couch and did not leave his home for 2 months because he feared he would float off into the clouds. We revisit Shane's therapy process at the end of this chapter.

In the sections below, we describe the sensory journey of external sensory input from the environment, known as exteroception, followed by how sensory input from the body is transmitted to the brain to facilitate interoception.

How the Brain Makes Sense of the World

Exteroception constitutes our ability to gather, process, and interpret information from the outside world, forming our perception of stimuli originating from the external environment. This mainly includes visual, acoustic, tactile, gustatory, and olfactory stimuli, while also extending to vestibular and proprioceptive stimuli in considering that gravity and objects felt by our muscles are external to the body. In this chapter, we aim to broadly determine how omnipresent exteroceptive sensory information is transmitted from the outside world to the brain and eventually enters our stream of consciousness.

Sensations that originate from stimuli outside the body and that are detected by the skin, ears, mouth, and eyes are transmitted to the brainstem in the survival brain, the lowest layer of the brain. Within the brainstem lies the reticular formation, which stems from the Latin word *reticulum*, meaning "net," and forms the basis of the RAS (Horn, 2006). The RAS acts similarly to a fishing net, where it catches a multitude of incoming input from the body and environment and acts to excite our arousal once stimuli are "caught." It spans the entire brainstem, mediating complex interactions between neurotransmitters involved in arousal and sleep–wake transition states (Routtenberg, 1968). At this level, the collective role of the RAS is to regulate autonomic function, muscle reflexes, and tone via descending reticulospinal (reticular formation to spinal cord) nerve pathways (see Table 2.1).

TABLE 2.1. Notable Brain Regions for Sensory Processing in the Brain

Brain area	Location	Function
Reticular activating system (RAS) • Ascending branch • Descending branch	Survival brain	• Plays a critical role in alertness and gatekeeping of information that enters our mainstream awareness • Ascending branch receives sensory signals from the body. • Descending branch is behaviorally driven, modulating muscle tone and initiating movements and postural changes.
Thalamus • Intralaminar nuclei	Emotional learning brain	• Acts as a sensory gateway that receives sensory information from the RAS and transmits it to specialized areas in the reflective brain
Ventral attention network • Ventral prefrontal cortex • Temporoparietal junction	Reflective brain	• Attentional network dedicated to bottom-up-driven sensory signals • Involved in environmental and internal monitoring
Dorsal attention network • Intraparietal sulcus • Frontal and supplemental eye fields	Reflective brain	• Voluntary orienting to visuospatial environment • Top-down, goal-oriented network
Primary visual cortex and visual association cortex (occipital lobe)	Reflective brain	• Awareness of visual stimuli • Analyzes color, depth, motion, and objects, including faces
Primary auditory cortex (temporal lobe)	Reflective brain	• Awareness of auditory stimuli • Processes complex auditory characteristics, like pitch and frequency • Language comprehension
Primary gustatory cortex (insula)	Reflective brain	• Central hub for processing taste • Overlaps with interoceptive processing hub
Primary sensory cortex	Reflective brain	• Contains sensory homunculus, a map of brain areas dedicated to somatosensory processing for different anatomical divisions of the body
Olfactory cortex	Emotional learning/ reflective brain	• Smell is relayed from the olfactory bulb (smell receptors) • Directly linked to emotional learning and memories via entorhinal cortex (hippocampus) and amygdala

Notably, the RAS also receives input from the periaqueductal gray in the survival brain, which is responsible for generating raw primal emotions, making the RAS–periaqueductal gray juncture a neural processing hub where arousal meets affect and sensation (Martins & Tavares, 2017).

Broadly, the RAS can be separated into two branches: descending and ascending. The descending RAS projects to the spinal cord in the form of postural changes initiated by the startle response or defensive posturing (e.g., fight-or-flight response), such as Jeremy's protective stance in response to background sensations while playing with his children in a park. The ascending RAS plays a vital role in wakefulness, as it acts as a gatekeeper for what we perceive in our consciousness as worthy of attention. Visceral sensations from the body are largely conveyed through the vagus and glossopharyngeal (mouth and throat) nerves; somatosensory pathways carrying mechanoreceptive input from the organs and viscera; and the splanchnic (abdominal cavity), phrenic (diaphragm), and cardiac (heart) nerves that travel through the spinal cord (Berthoud & Neuhuber, 2000; Cramer & Darby, 2014). These act as key conduits for the brain–body connection and are instrumental for connecting our body to our state of consciousness. For example, "a sudden pit in your stomach" can help direct your attention to perceived danger. The persistent visceral feeling of doom leads Jeremy to always be hypervigilant to sensations in his surroundings, where his conscious awareness is always consumed by mostly irrelevant sensations. By contrast, an internal sense of calmness and relaxation takes us out of a state of hyperarousal, frees up our cognitive resources, and allows us to safely connect with others and feel a sense of belonging: an elusive and rare experience for traumatized individuals.

Sensory information that enters the RAS is eventually transmitted to the intralaminar nuclei of the thalamus in the emotional learning brain (Yeo, Chang, & Jang, 2013), from which it travels to the reflective brain to guide conscious decision making (Table 2.1). In other words, it allows for a filtering of sensory information to help the brain determine what is most important to spend energy attending to. Particularly, the thalamus acts as a "sensory gateway" connecting the RAS and specialized areas in the reflective brain that are integral for sensory integration, or the higher-level organization and interpretation of a combination of sensory inputs (Ayres, 1972). This process also influences the connection between the thalamus and other brain areas involved in higher-order functions, like attention, agency of movement, and perception of a unified sensory experience. Thus, the thalamus acts as a unique conduit that connects the survival brain layer with upper specialized layers of the reflective brain to direct attention to sensory events and facilitate alertness. Alertness can be defined as a state of active attention characterized by high sensory awareness—thus, a greater level of alertness would require increased employment of attentional processes in the reflective brain. In Jeremy's case, his visceral sense of impending doom creates a persistent hyperaroused state where he is overattentive to exteroceptive stimuli, ranging from the sight of falling leaves to the crackling sound of fireworks.

The reflective brain operates largely through neural networks, or brain structures working in tandem, that give rise to the dynamic and rich experience of being human. While these neural networks are covered more extensively in Chapters 6 and 8, we here highlight the dorsal and ventral attention networks as they are involved in navigating sensory and emotional stimuli in the environment (Seeley et al., 2007). The ventral attention network includes the ventral prefrontal cortex and the TPJ and is involved with responding to bottom-up sensory stimulation. Its counterpart, the dorsal attention network, comprises the intraparietal sulcus in the parietal lobe and the frontal eye fields and is known for *voluntarily* orienting one's visuospatial attention. This is a top-down function that is consciously goal directed and intentional rather than a subconscious response to environmental signals (Farrant & Uddin, 2015; Vossel, Geng, & Fink, 2014). This attentional bifurcation into ventral and dorsal attention networks forms a unique dynamic to mediate top-down goals with bottom-up processing, making them putative targets for interventions focused on shifting one's responses to trauma-related stimuli. In Shane's case, the exteroceptive tactile sensations evoked during his unsuccessful restraint therapy became associated with intense visceral sensations related to powerlessness and shame. This associated visceral-affective experience made Shane unable to engage attentively with his environment and caused him to feel withdrawn while his motor tics became further exacerbated. This association illustrates how specific sensations can be intricately linked to emotional and behavioral states, where sensations from our past are emotionally evocative and affect how we allocate our attentional resources. For Jeremy, the crackling sound of fireworks or the rustling of leaves initiated a strong bottom-up ventral attention network response associated with a paralyzing fear from past rocket attacks, directing his neural resources toward frantically protecting himself and his family.

While the ventral attention network receives sensations from the environment, the following sensations are also processed at higher-order areas in the reflective brain via the thalamus (the vestibular and interoceptive senses are explored in more depth in Chapters 5 and 6, respectively):

• Visual sensations are processed in the occipital lobe toward the back of the brain. While the primary visual cortex in the occipital lobe is responsible for our awareness of visual stimuli (Murray et al., 2016), the visual association cortex that spans the occipital lobe allows for a complex analysis of visual stimuli, such as understanding and recognizing visual sensations from the past and interpreting their various characteristics, including object, color, depth, and motion (Bak et al., 1990). Notably, the fusiform gyrus in the occipital lobe is associated with facial recognition and has been previously shown to maintain direct connections with the periaqueductal gray in the survival brain section (Harricharan et al., 2016; McCarthy, Puce, Gore, & Allison, 1997). This may be why viewing faces similar to those from traumatic experiences can elicit arousal and raw emotional responses at the same intensity as was experienced at the time of the trauma.

- Auditory information is processed in the temporal lobe of the brain, and it allows for analyzing complex sounds as well as discerning language, pitch, and prosody (Byron & Alfredo, 2016; Devlin et al., 2003). Toward the back of the temporal lobe lies Wernicke's area, which is heavily involved in language comprehension (DeWitt & Rauschecker, 2013).

- Gustatory (taste) information is processed in the gustatory cortex, located in the insula of the reflective brain. Thus, gustatory processing has substantial overlap with the central processing hub for interoceptive visceral sensations (Veldhuizen et al., 2011). The gustatory cortex allows for complex analysis of various taste characteristics (e.g., bitter, salty, sour, umami, or sweet).

- Smell information travels through the most unique neural pathway for sensory processing in the brain as it directly enters the reflective brain via the olfactory bulb, bypassing sensory transmission through the thalamus of the emotional learning brain and RAS of the survival brain (Mombaerts, 2001). Critically, the olfactory bulb is directly linked to the amygdala and the hippocampus, key structures in the emotional learning brain that are also involved with storing memories (Wilson & Stevenson, 2003). The olfactory bulb's proximity to the brain's emotion and memory centers helps explain why certain scents can immediately trigger a vivid memory associated with a strong emotion.

- Somatosensory information from the skin and internal body is processed in the postcentral gyrus, commonly referred to as the primary sensory cortex, which acts as the first reflective brain-level processing center for somatosensory input (Ploner, Schmitz, Freund, & Schnitzler, 2000), which we discuss more in depth below.

In order for somatosensory information from the external world to reach the brain, the receptors on our skin need to send information (action potentials) through tracts, or bundles of nerve fibers, up the spinal cord to arrive at the survival brain (Preusser et al., 2015). Some information from these skin receptors initiates subconscious responses where we need to act without thinking, such as modulating defensive motor responses to threat. As Plate 2.1 shows, somatosensory information heavily innervates numerous regions in the survival brain that help carry out these defensive motor responses, including the RAS, cerebellum, vestibular nuclei, periaqueductal gray, and superior colliculus (Ferrè & Haggard, 2015; Harricharan et al., 2016; Olivé, Tempelmann, Berthoz, & Heinze, 2015). Thus, it is critical to consider the contributions that somatosensory information provides to the survival brain functioning, as well as its further cascading effects on the emotional and reflective brain layers. These tracts transmit tactile sensory information through the thalamus to the primary sensory cortex to help us consciously navigate the external world.

The primary sensory cortex (S1) in the reflective brain also acts as a map for how sensory information is perceived from different areas of the body (Table 2.1).

The S1 surface area dedicated to a particular part of the body is proportional to the density of somatosensory receptors in that specific region (Muret, Root, Kieliba, Clode, & Makin, 2022; Roux, Djidjeli, & Durand, 2018). In other words, areas of the body with greater and more complex interactions are more largely represented in the brain map of the primary sensory cortex, whereas areas that are less often used make up smaller proportions of the map. For example, the hands, lips, and face make up larger proportions of the brain map due to their frequency of use in our day-to-day life. S1 contains a somatotopic map, or *sensory homunculus*, where the parts of the body are presented in an organized fashion. The top of the homunculus starts with the anatomical lower half of the body (e.g., toes, foot, leg, hip) and progressively moves up the body as you go farther down the homunculus. The lowest portion of the homunculus represents our facial exteroceptive receptors, including the eye, nose, face, and tongue. Importantly, recent research has shown that the homunculus contains interspersed emotional hubs, highlighting the inextricable link between sensory and emotional processing (Giraud et al., 2024; see Figure 2.1).

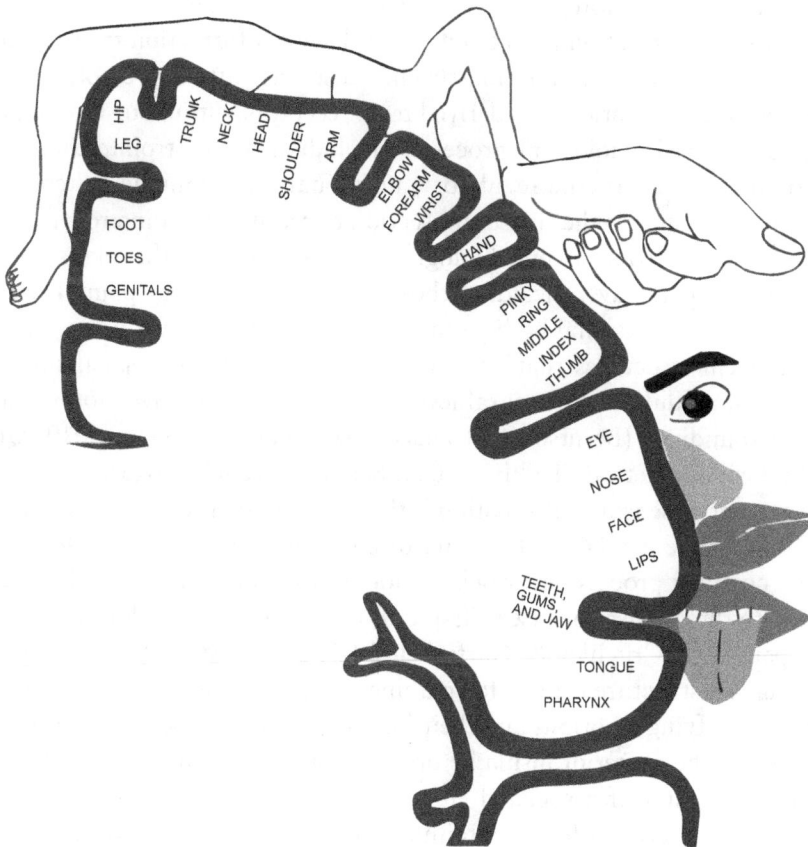

FIGURE 2.1. Visual depiction of the sensory homunculus.

Sensations Foster Emotion

In Chapter 1, we discussed how sensory information travels through the brain, with sensory information from the outside world interacting with sensations experienced within the body to guide our understanding of and reactions to our surroundings. As previously mentioned, various sources of sensory information enter the survival brain first. Here, neural pathways are influenced by the emotional *valence* of incoming sensory information, or its positive or negative emotional coloring relative to context (Rachman, 1980).

When external sources of sensory information enter the survival brain, they are accompanied by interoceptive (visceral) sensations, which help determine the emotional valence of the incoming external input (Critchley & Garfinkel, 2017; Harricharan et al., 2021; Wiens, 2005). Again, consider holding a loved one's hand while walking outside. The tactile receptors in the palm of your hand will be activated, leading to a feeling of warmth, connection, and belonging. Then, imagine holding the hand of somebody who has hurt you in the past. While the sources of sensory input remain the same, they can elicit profoundly different emotions, such as fear or terror. Therefore, it is imperative to understand how the context within which sensory information is received can influence information transfer through sensory-based pathways and ultimately elicit distinctly different emotions.

Interoceptive sensations are derived from receptors within our internal organs and driven by basic biological processes, including the gastrointestinal, cardiovascular, respiratory, thermoregulatory, hormonal, and immune systems (Craig, 2003). The brainstem is the first brain section to receive direct interoceptive information ascending from visceral biological systems through the vagus nerve and somatosensory pathways, including those that detect visceral pain (Paciorek & Skora, 2020). Once internal bodily sensations reach the survival brain, they influence brainstem structures that are wired to maintain physiological functioning via the ANS, modulate our arousal level, and initiate instinctive motor responses to our surroundings (Berntson & Khalsa, 2021; Paulus & Stein, 2010; Quigley, Kanoski, Grill, Barrett, & Tsakiris, 2021; Schulz & Vogele, 2015).

Interoceptive sensory information is then relayed via the thalamus in the emotional brain to the insula and the anterior cingulate cortex in the reflective brain for more complex processing, which is thought to help identify or label the emotions tied to these sensations (see Chapter 6 for an in-depth exploration of interoceptive pathways; Critchley & Garfinkel, 2017; Zaki, Davis, & Ochsner, 2012). The insula is a structure critical for making sense of these inner "gut" sensations and thus identifying emotions and their intensity. Raw interoceptive sensory input first travels to the posterior insula before traversing to the anterior insula for conscious identification of associated emotional labels (Wiens, 2005). Notably, the anterior insula is crucial for maintaining one's sense of time and understanding the chronology of events (Craig, 2009; Simmons et al., 2013) to better inform how these sensations are interpreted. For example, if an individual gets into an intense argument with someone else, the process may go as follows:

- They are likely to start feeling their inner body temperature rising and their heart rate increasing.
- These interoceptive sensations stemming from the inner body are initially relayed to the brainstem to elicit a preconscious reaction at the level of the periaqueductal gray (Berntson & Khalsa, 2021).
- From here, the ANS is activated to regulate heart and respiration rates and initiate defensive behaviors that react to what transpired during the argument (e.g., forming fists with your hands; Tsakiris, Tajadura-Jimenez, & Costantini, 2011).
- Afterward, this sensory input may be sent to the insula to help identify anger as a primary emotion underpinning these visceral and somatic sensations. The insula also aids in determining the level of anger one feels, as well as detecting the amount of time elapsed while feeling these sensations.
- Ideally, this information is eventually relayed to the prefrontal cortex in the reflective brain to guide the best course of action in response to the argument, imbued with insights from past experience and social norms.

We must experience a sensation in order to remember it; sensory experiences are the building blocks that form the foundation for memories of the past (Damasio, 1998; Ianì, 2019; Kearney & Lanius, 2024). This "current sensation" to the "past memory" pipeline ultimately allows us to recall how the body had previously responded to sensations and informs an appropriate response in the future. For example, you may pass by your favorite coffee shop and anticipate the taste, smell, and warmth of your regular coffee order. This sensory imprint may have occurred alongside positive experiences, such as an increased body temperature on a cold February afternoon and enhanced focus at work for the rest of the day. Your ability to anticipate the sensory–emotional inputs that coincide with past experiences is quite adaptive, in that it allows you to familiarize yourself with positive and negative sensory experiences and plan your actions accordingly.

Substantial energy expenditure is required to attend to new sensory experiences given that your brain and body are forced to come up with a measured reaction (Quigley et al., 2021). The human body has evolved to imprint these internal sensory experiences into our brains through a process called *interoceptive predicting*, where we preconsciously monitor inner bodily signals rather than expending energy to respond to each sensory experience at the level of the reflective brain (Marshall, Gentsch, & Schutz-Bosbach, 2018; Owens, Allen, Ondobaka, & Friston, 2018; Seth & Friston, 2016). This is how internal organ systems within our body function, where humans instinctively know what to do to manage physiological sensations like hunger, thirst, or bladder fullness. These sensations do not require additional complex functioning, thereby allowing interoceptive predictions to help the body conserve energy (Marshall et al., 2018; Owens et al., 2018; Seth & Friston, 2016). By contrast, feeling an unanticipated knot in your stomach while watching current world news can reach higher brain sections that lead to more complex mental and behavioral adaptations to make meaning of these unexpected sensations, which cannot be accomplished at an automatic level (see Chapter 6). Together, interoceptive predictions and higher brain functions let us meet the demands of our inner and outer environments.

In the aftermath of trauma, the survival brain is in overdrive, where dysregulated arousal and autonomic responses lead to difficulties processing incoming sensory input (Harricharan et al., 2020; Paulus & Stein, 2010). The brain's receipt of a continuous stream of inner visceral sensations may elicit very different reactions after trauma. Since traumatic memories encode their own unique sensory imprints, interoceptive imprints like pain and temperature from these memories may also be subjected to interoceptive predictive coding (Seth, Suzuki, & Critchley, 2012). If an individual experienced raw, visceral sensations of pain and temperature during a traumatic event, they may associate any new sensations of pain and temperature with prominent trauma-related emotions like guilt, shame, and anger. In other words, emotions rooted in trauma can be pervasive because they are continuously reinforced by inner visceral sensations, creating an internal feedback loop. For Shane, revisited below, any touch or movements outside of his control elicited accompanying feelings of visceral distress and shame. These shame-related emotions that became associated with incoming somatosensory, vestibular, or visceral sensations were due to the interoceptive predictions his brain had developed based on past sensory–emotional associations. Thus, any subsequent experience of restraint drew on his previous interoceptive predictions fueling panic, terror, and/ or shame. This feedback loop reinforces the relationship between sensations and trauma-related emotions, leading to consequent avoidance of vital daily activities.

To harness neuroplasticity and retrain the interoceptive coding maps in the brain, sensory-guided exercises can be used to break these inner feedback loops and create new sensory imprints that reframe the interoceptive predictions in the body. For example, if physical pleasure from endorphins is coded in the brain as shameful after trauma, the objective would be to shift this prediction toward joy through discovery of novel, safe sensations in the context of a secure therapeutic relationship. Here, increasing an awareness of bodily sensations in a guided, safe manner can help shift the locus of control from the survival brain toward the reflective brain, ultimately leading to greater unity among brain, mind, and body. Below, we revisit Shane's journey through his therapeutic process to highlight the importance of reassociating sensations with positive emotions and empowering experiences.

Revisiting Shane: The Sensory Pathway to Healing

Shane's psychiatrist eventually encouraged his parents to seek interdisciplinary treatment involving an occupational therapist to help rehabilitate his functioning to allow him to participate in the basic activities of daily living. At the start of treatment, Shane moved as one with his couch: any time a part of his body did not touch it, he would start to tic unless it was to fulfill the primal human need of going to the bathroom. Once his therapist understood that he needed to meet

Shane where he was, they started achieving small milestones. For the first time, this created a kernel of hope for recovery in Shane's treatment. At the start of every session, the therapist would offer opportunities to engage in gentle vestibular and proprioceptive experiences to restore his sense of connection to and agency over his body. For example, the therapist brought a Lycra rope and played tug-of-war, explicitly having Shane set the pace. This allowed Shane to regain some semblance of control over his body, which was progressively lost during his traumatic experiences in the hospital. One day, while engaging in back-and-forth movements with his therapist using the Lycra rope, Shane stood up for the first time in months. When this breakthrough occurred, Shane had a burst of tics, jumped back down onto the couch, and curled up into a ball due to this unfamiliar experience.

An exchange between Shane and his therapist follows.

SHANE (S): (*Tics vocally.*)

THERAPIST (T): What is it? (*Inquires curiously.*)

S: I stood up (*looks excited*), but my tics are back (*face saddens*).

T: How did it feel?

S: It's the first time I've done it for something else other than going to the bathroom. It feels good.

T: Do you want to try the game again?

S: I'm not sure. I'm scared.

T: How about we start from where you are, and we go from there? You are already sitting on the edge of the couch. We don't even have to stand up.

S: Okay.

The therapist's respect for Shane's individual pace allowed him to feel safe enough to engage in more movement activities with the therapist, such as jumping on a trampoline. One step eventually led to 10 steps. He started to move around his living room, which expanded to his backyard, then a park, then finally back to school. Shane's journey was not over following his occupational therapy sessions. He was reminded of his traumatic experience any time he stepped into a hospital for his regular checkups and endured relapses at home before and after these visits. Although his tics were still present, he saw them as part of his uniqueness and not as a disability. By age 17, he finished high school, worked internships, and for the first time in years, started to contemplate a future life worth living.

One of the final exchanges between Shane and his therapist follows:

S: I'd like to help people with Tourette's when I'm older. Do you think I can do it?

T: (*Playfully*) It is not what I think that matters; it's whatever you think is possible! I think you are capable of anything.

S: (*Smiles.*)

The battlefield that was once Shane's home eventually became his peaceful haven.

Putting It All Together

The journey of sensory information through the brain is vital for our ability to interpret and interact with the world effectively. The aftermath of trauma can leave individuals susceptible to alterations regarding how sensations are interpreted in the brain, thereby disrupting one's capacity for emotion regulation. This can beget the instinctual emergence of raw visceral emotions that are difficult to temper without the necessary higher-order processing from cortical structures in the reflective brain. As demonstrated in Shane's case, understanding the interplay between sensory processing and emotions posttrauma is essential for developing effective therapeutic interventions and supporting recovery. These approaches often incorporate sensory-based interventions to help individuals regain a sense of control and stability. For example, incorporating calming sensory experiences, such as rhythmic play or mindful exposure to specific sounds or textures, can promote the discovery of safe sensations and reinforce sensory pathways that incorporate all three sections of the brain. When the reflective brain is in dynamic engagement with the lower sections of the brain, it can build more sensory awareness and emotional resilience through the new association of safe sensations with more positively valenced emotions. An increased sensory awareness can significantly enhance social engagement by fostering a deeper connection to both our own experiences and those of others. Being mindful of our own sensory experiences helps us articulate our needs and emotions more clearly, promoting more introspection about the meaning of the past, and may even encourage more reciprocal exchanges with others. Shane was able to reclaim his sense of belonging in both his body and the world after therapy, where he gradually regained the capacity to feel alive as an active participant in his daily life. In Bridging to Practice 2, we offer strategies to help diversify our sensory palettes to allow discovery of both safe and unsafe sensations—such as noticing the nuances in tone of voice, the subtleties of body language, or the emotional impact of different environments—which can foster a transformational shift toward unifying the mind, brain, and body.

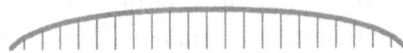

BRIDGING TO PRACTICE 2
Tuning In to Safe Sensations

The genius of the traumatized brain is its ability to adapt to inescapable threat to maximize chances of survival. Here, it becomes a master at quickly detecting unsafe sensations from within the body and from the external environment. The traumatized brain learns to predict that threat is inevitable and anticipates unsafe sensory input at any moment. Any bodily sensation or sensory input from the environment remotely reminiscent of previous traumatic experiences is registered by the survival brain as unsafe at a preconscious level. Even though these are incredibly adaptive means of coping with the horror of trauma, they come at a cost: *The traumatized individual is left not fully knowing what feeling safe is like.* In fact, when feelings of safety are unknown, unpredictability and chaos feel like home. Frequently, the brain and body do not know what safe sensations feel like—such experiences often taken for granted are experienced as foreign entities. What do sensations of loving and nurturing touch feel like? What is it like to experience the soothing voice of a supportive other? What is it like to experience being held by another through a supportive gaze? And finally, what is it like to engage in a soothing rocking motion alone or with another?

Introducing the traumatized brain and body to safe sensations is critical in setting the stage for recovery. Here, it is crucial that sensations of safety need to be introduced slowly since they can be extremely overwhelming for the traumatized individual who often has only known sensations associated with threat. Asking your client to identify "what sensation is your body seeking to make you feel safer" can be an important first step in helping the client to become curious and aware about what safe sensations their system is seeking. This is also a crucial process for helping your client feel safe and grounded in the present. Allow ample time for the client to tune in to what they need. Believe in your clients! They have incredible knowledge and wisdom, which frequently feels very inaccessible to them. The therapeutic relationship provides the anchor for the client to explore safe sensory input.

Taking Small Steps toward Tuning In to Safe Sensations

1. Form a trusting relationship to build an anchor for the client to explore safe sensory input.

2. Provide psychoeducation about how the brain and body have adapted to focus on sensations of threat to survive at the expense of safe sensations.

3. Help the client to become more and more aware of what sensations are triggering for them (bodily sensations and sensations from the external environment).

4. Help the client to understand that becoming used to safe sensations is critical to feel grounded in and safe in the present.

5. Check in with the client about what it is like for them to think about becoming used to experiencing safe sensations and starting to think about feeling safe. Be aware that the word *safe* can be triggering for some individuals. If this is the case, ask the client what word would be more suitable for them.

6. Reassure the client that they are in control of the pace of therapy. Remember, the slower you go, the faster you get there!

7. Slowly begin to identify safe sensations with the client. Ask them, "What sensation is your body seeking to make you feel safer?" Reassure them that all the answers are within them, and that the therapist functions as a coach who will help them access their inner wisdom.

For example, in our experience, clients have identified many different sensations associated with safety:

Visual

   a. Looking at a picture of an animal or a safe person
   b. Focusing on something that feels safe in a room

Auditory

   a. Listening to different types of music depending on the client's arousal and emotional state
   b. Listening to sounds of nature (e.g., sitting by the water)

Olfactory

   a. Smelling different types of essential oils
   b. Smelling blossoming trees or fresh flowers

Taste

   a. Focusing on the taste of a strong flavor (this may vary depending on the person's arousal and emotional state)
   b. Drinking herbal tea

Touch

   a. Holding a pillow close to their abdomen and chest
   b. Touching a soft object
   c. Rubbing the hand on sandpaper
   d. Rubbing an ice cube on the arm
   e. Taking a cold shower

Proprioceptive

   a. Using a weighted blanket
   b. Using a body sock
   c. Crunching ice or food to give proprioceptive input to the jaw

Vestibular

   a. Gently rocking back and forth on a rocking chair
   b. Orienting eyes to a safe object in the room

Interoceptive

    a. Feeling sensations of tenderness when looking at a picture of an animal

    b. Feeling sensations of awe when immersed in nature

8. Ask your client to notice what they feel inside before and after seeking a sensation that feels safe for them.

9. Remind your client that they are seeking different sensations depending on the arousal and emotional state of the individual.

10. Work with the client to create a toolkit consisting of different sensations they can use to create safety.

11. Have faith in your client! In time, they will be able to tune into what safe sensations their body is seeking.

3

Feeling Safe or Under Threat

THE DIVERGING ROADS OF SENSORY EXPERIENCE

An adventure is only an inconvenience rightly considered.
An inconvenience is only an adventure wrongly considered.
—G. K. Chesterton

Incoming sensory information from our surroundings and body enters the survival brain at the level of the superior colliculus and the periaqueductal gray, respectively. As outlined in Chapter 1, both structures are located in the midbrain, a portion of the survival brain that sits between the brainstem and the emotional brain. The superior colliculus and the periaqueductal gray are intimately connected. While the superior colliculus is a site of low-level multisensory integration, the periaqueductal gray is where sensory information and its concomitant arousal response meets raw positive and negative emotion, including FEAR, RAGE, CARE, SEEK, LUST, PANIC, and PLAY (Panksepp, 2004).

Based on the integration of sensory and raw emotional information, the survival brain coordinates the most appropriate response. These innate responses spare us from needing to recruit the emotional or reflective brain sections, which would take up precious time and preclude a swift response to imminent threat. Various instinctual defensive reactions are mediated by the deep layers of the superior colliculus and periaqueductal gray, including fleeing, fighting, freezing/tonic immobility, and emotional shutdown. The latter two responses result in either muscles being locked in position to avoid motion detection by a predator or flaccid muscle tone to feign death in the face of an imminent predator (Bandler, Keay, Floyd, & Price, 2000; Kozlowska et al., 2015; Lanius et al., 2017; Mobbs et al., 2007; Schauer & Elbert, 2010; Terpou, Densmore, et al., 2019). For example, some patients describe feeling as though their entire body or parts of their body are "encased in cement" when faced with a trigger.

The superior colliculus and the periaqueductal gray are extremely efficient at reacting with the most appropriate defensive response for our survival outside our conscious control. In fact, the survival brain can initiate sudden defensive reactions in less than 20 milliseconds, as opposed to more than 100 milliseconds from the reflective brain (Chen, Yaseen, Cohen, & Hallett, 1998). It is important to note that the survival brain also has the ability to process sight, sound, and touch beneath our conscious awareness.

Alternatively, if the incoming sensory–emotional information signals *safety*, the survival brain takes full advantage of the reflective brain's capacity to do a more thorough evaluation of the incoming sensory–emotional information and interpret the context of these sensations. At the reflective brain, we can become fully aware and reflect on the sensory information of our external and internal worlds, plan appropriate responses, and consciously connect with others in regard to their intentions and perspectives.

Threat versus Safety

Let us look at an example to illustrate how the survival brain operates. Imagine going on a walk with a loved one. You are holding hands, feeling a sense of belonging and love for each other while enjoying the beautiful scenery around you. The scent of gas and a high-pitched noise makes you turn your head and neck to locate an oncoming truck, which is coming to a stop. As you are about to cross the road with your loved one, the truck suddenly starts to accelerate, causing you to startle. Here, you are forced to react very quickly without thinking or being fully aware of the situation to get you and your loved one to safety. You instinctively pull yourself and your loved one to the sidewalk. After, you may experience fear or rage at the reckless driver and begin to feel your heart racing, your palms sweating, and a knot in your stomach, realizing you could have died. These reactions occur through the periaqueductal gray's connections with the sympathetic nervous system and emotional brain. As you start to realize the magnitude of what transpired, you slowly realize that you reacted automatically and reflexively to the threat of your loved one being hurt—without thinking about it or consciously planning your response. This can incur a breakdown in communication between the three sections of the brain responsible for sensory processing, which leads to *sensory disintegration*, where the experience cannot be processed as a whole.

Let us consider this example again, but under conditions of safety. Again, imagine going for a walk and crossing the road with a loved one. You are again holding hands, feeling a sense of belonging and love for each other while enjoying the beauty of nature around you. The scent of gas makes you turn your head to orient toward the oncoming truck. You see the truck stopped at the intersection and therefore decide to cross the road together. This time, the truck remains stationary as you safely cross the road, all the while laughing together as you tell a funny story. You are able to sense the visceral comfort and joy from this shared experience, feel the warmth of the springtime sun, and see the beauty of the flowering trees around you. This is an example of incoming sensory–emotional information signaling safety and trust at the level of the survival brain. Under these conditions, the survival brain can facilitate *sensory integration*: It connects optimally with the emotional learning and the reflective brain sections to interpret the sensory information of our external and internal worlds, move with intention, connect on a conscious level, and later feel warmth when recalling this sweet moment in your personal history (see Plate 3.1 for an illustration).

How the Traumatized Brain Reacts to the World

How is it, then, that traumatized individuals so often misinterpret sensory–emotional inputs as threats? Revisiting the above example in a traumatized person may illustrate the profound effect that trauma can have on how we perceive our internal and external worlds. In crossing the road, the traumatized individual may already be hypervigilant. Negotiating the outside world feels frequently terrifying as their hypervigilance creates a profound sensitivity to almost every sensation encountered in the environment. They detect headlights in their periphery and, although the truck does come to a stop, grab their partner and vigorously move them out of the road regardless. Their heart rate and breathing rate accelerate and remain elevated for nearly 10 minutes as they sit on the curb and try to regain their bearings. They feel incredibly misunderstood by their confused partner who attempts to comfort them. The traumatized individual's sense of belonging and love from their partner frequently feels dulled on the backdrop of having been chronically emotionally hurt and misunderstood by their caregiver early in life. They view the world as an unsafe place, constantly anticipating danger and impending doom, thus preventing them from fully experiencing and discovering beauty and social connection. The negative perception of the external world is further fueled by painful internal sensations and inner bodily tension, such as generalized muscle tension and feeling their stomach as permanently in a knot. Unbeknownst to the individual, they are feeling the effects of *sensory disintegration* across the three sections of the brain. The survival brain seems to be on overdrive, working overtime never to miss a beat again.

The traumatized individual's inner experiences can often swing like a pendulum from one extreme to another, from gut-wrenching inner tension to emotional detachment or numbness. One moment, it is gnawing sensations that feel as though they are threatened and being eaten up alive inside—the next moment, it is emotional numbness and flatness. The latter states, as first described by Pierre Janet (1889), are frequently accompanied by the absence of feeling either pleasure or pain and are associated with an inner lifelessness, or feeling "dead inside" (van der Kolk, Brown, & van der Hart, 1989). Henry Krystal (1988), who survived the Holocaust, labeled his experience with numbing as "emotional anesthesia" and noted:

> The paradox in the traumatic state is that the numbing and closing off are experienced as relief from the previously painful affect such as anxiety; at the same time, they are also experienced as the first part of dying, for, along with the affective blocking, there is a blocking of initiative and all life-preserving cognition. (p. 151)

Furthermore, any external sensations from the environment are commonly experienced by the traumatized individual as hostile to the point of feeling like the world is no longer a safe place. The traumatized person is often observed in a hypervigilant state, constantly scanning the environment for dangerous cues. In essence, many sensory cues in the environment have become a potential source of danger, where the traumatized brain has difficulty distinguishing safe versus threatening sensations. This difficulty leads to a close monitoring of the environment at all times.

If this state becomes too intense and persists for too long, the traumatized individual can become detached from their inner and outer worlds, diminishing or shutting down sensory input as a means for survival in a chronically overwhelmed, unbearable state of vulnerability. This shutting down has been proposed to be associated with sensory information being trapped at the level of the thalamus, a central relay station in the emotional learning brain that facilitates connection between the survival brain and the reflective brain sections to provide integration and context to sensory information (for review, see Lanius et al., 2017). This process has been defined in the neuroscientific literature as thalamocortical deafferentation (Krystal, 1995). This could indicate that sensory experiences become locked in the survival and emotional learning brain sections. They are thus inaccessible to the reflective self, which is critical to knowing what we feel (Plate 3.1).

Under these conditions of chronic threat, the survival brain does not optimally connect with the emotional and reflective brain sections (Harricharan et al., 2020; Lanius et al., 2017; Mobbs et al., 2009) to take advantage of the brain's full capacities. With its propensity for eliciting swift defensive responses, the survival brain often runs the show. This comes at the expense of being able to reflect upon and learn from one's experience, all the while diminishing our ability to feel fully alive in connection with ourselves and the world around us. Indeed, feeling constantly and imminently threatened propagates and amplifies sensory processing predominantly at the survival brain, which sustains a lower level of consciousness (Panksepp, 2004). This lower level of consciousness maximizes fast, reflexive responding not only to react quickly without thinking but also to conserve energy for survival. This differs markedly from processing sensory information in reflective brain structures that are critical for higher levels of consciousness, including intentional movements/agency, language, social connection, and mentalizing the emotional states of our loved ones. These processes require significantly more energy than activation of lower survival brain structures.

Shifting and adapting brain activation to lower-level survival brain structures therefore comes at the cost of *sensory integration*: integrating our senses into the reflective cortical brain, where we can orient our awareness to the present moment. Instead, the trauma survivor is often in a state of *sensory disintegration*: feeling like the past has become the present, where the survival brain takes the driver's seat in preparation for any potential repeat of the horrifying past. As a result, critical aspects of a fully functioning sense of self, including agency, reflection, curiosity, and social connection are severely compromised.

How the Body Remembers: Memories Are Connected to the Senses

Memory is the process through which we retain information over time. Human memory uses past experiences, inclusive of their associated sensations, emotions, and actions, to help guide how we navigate toward the future. It organizes and stores event-related information, allowing individuals to recall and draw upon past events to develop an understanding of the world within the present. The elusive neurobiological underpinnings of human memory have been an area of robust and evolving research that remains inconclusive to this day. Current trends in neuroscience research suggest that memory formation occurs through continual modifications to communication patterns among specific cells, called engram cells, that can change and hold information based on specific experiences (Ortega-de San Luis, Pezzoli, Urrieta, & Ryan, 2023). It is thought that the transfer of information between these engram cells gives rise to the retrieval of past experiences, further strengthening the idea that neuroplasticity is based on ongoing modifications to neuronal communication.

Three main processes characterize memory: encoding, storage, and retrieval. First, encoding refers to the process through which information is learned (Tulving & Thomson, 1973). This is facilitated by all the human sensory systems (Beiser & Houk, 1998; Kayser, Ince, & Panzeri, 2012). This sensory information is combined to create a multisensory perspective that interacts with the brain's memory networks to understand the meaning of incoming sensory information in light of past experiences (Quak, London, & Talsma, 2015; Shams & Seitz, 2008). Sleep plays a central role in memory encoding as it helps to solidify memories through a process called consolidation (Diekelmann, Wilhelm, & Born, 2009; Rothschild, 2019; Stickgold, 2005). Recent experiences are transformed into long-term memory during sleep, particularly when the brain enters the rapid eye movement (REM) phase of sleep (Siegel, 2001). The periaqueductal gray in the survival brain plays a critical role in the consolidation of memory as it helps to balance hormones important for sleep, including cortisol and melatonin, which in turn help regulate REM sleep cycles (Murkar & De Koninck, 2018; Peever & Fuller, 2017). The locus coeruleus, another survival brain structure involved in our stress response and arousal, is highly involved in our sleep–wake cycle and has been shown to reduce its firing during REM sleep (Takahashi, Kayama, Lin, & Sakai, 2010). This is to suggest that the survival brain is involved not only in sensory integration and survival responses but also in sleep–wake cycles critical for memory consolidation processes.

After encoding, memory is stored. Memory storage can be broken into short-term and long-term memory (Goelet, Castellucci, Schacher, & Kandel, 1986). Short-term memory, often referred to as working memory, is a transient memory process driven by the immediate, most salient sensory information that is required for attention (Angelopoulou & Drigas, 2021; Burgess & Hitch, 2006; Goelet et al., 1986). Long-term memory, however, leaves sensory imprints on the brain that hold personal meaning and are stored for retrieval in the future.

Finally, retrieval is the process through which individuals access this stored information through purposeful or cued remembrance (Baddeley, Lewis, Eldridge, & Thomson, 1984; Frankland, Josselyn, & Kohler, 2019; Williams & Hollan, 1981). Long-term memories are retrieved through association, such as driving past your former primary school and remembering a former teacher's name.

The autobiographical memory (memory of an individual's life events) framework involves multiple sections of the brain, including the emotional learning brain and the reflective brain (Spreng & Grady, 2010; Svoboda, McKinnon, & Levine, 2006). In particular, the hippocampus, a key brain region located in the emotional learning brain, is involved in autobiographical memory, future-oriented thinking, spatial memory, planning, and navigation (Addis, Moscovitch, Crawley, & McAndrews, 2004; Cabeza & St Jacques, 2007). The hippocampus has two subregions: the anterior hippocampus, which is theorized to be associated with emotional aspects of memory, and the posterior hippocampus, which is more involved with the spatial orientation and sensory aspects of memory (DeMaster, Pathman, Lee, & Ghetti, 2014; Poppenk & Moscovitch, 2011). Sensory imprints from long-term memory are retrieved from the posterior hippocampus and connections are formed with reflective brain regions to help guide behavior. Essentially, the hippocampus connects sensory and motor information from past experiences with present occurrences, facilitating learning and memory consolidation (Poppenk & Moscovitch, 2011).

Reliving, Not Remembering

The hippocampus's connections to higher cortical areas and therefore its role in memory processes can be affected among traumatized individuals, who are often plagued by intrusive memories and flashbacks from traumatic events (Clancy et al., 2024; Karl et al., 2006). It has been suggested that the posterior hippocampus can contribute to traumatized individuals' experience of *reliving* sensory details from traumatic memories, which is distinct from normal autobiographical memories that are *remembered* (Kearney & Lanius, 2024). Recent findings among individuals with PTSD suggest that the posterior hippocampus exhibits limited connections with key higher-reflective brain areas involved in orientation of the body in space, including the supramarginal gyrus, indicating that one's sense of body in space during traumatic memory retrieval may be disrupted (Chaposhloo et al., 2023). For example, if an individual was sexually assaulted while lying down, they may feel disconnected from their body when going to sleep due to the postural reminder of the trauma.

Pierre Janet (1889), a pioneer in understanding and treating PTSD, first suggested that memories of traumatic experiences are distinct from typical autobiographical memories because of their emotional salience, causing them to feel relived in the present. Over a century later, research is indeed finding that traumatic memory is a discrete phenomenon distinguishable from sad but nontraumatic autobiographical memory in areas such as the hippocampus (Perl et al., 2023). Brewin, Dalgleish, and Joseph (1996) further described the involuntary nature of reliving, while also suggesting that the intense, vivid sensory impressions characteristic of reliving result in a feeling of "nowness," creating a sense of timelessness. This sense of timelessness prevents one from acknowledging the traumatic event as an event from the past (see also van der Kolk & Fisler, 1995; van der Kolk & van der Hart, 1991).

There is now ample evidence to suggest that involuntary reliving of traumatic memories through flashbacks stems from intense sensory imprints that are encoded in a fragmented manner. This fragmentation then leads to poorly contextualized memories that are difficult to process (Brewin, 2014). Moreover, decreased capacity to encode sensorimotor sensations from traumatic memories can disrupt the brain's sensorimotor network, a group of brain regions involved in sensorimotor processing and motor action. The sensorimotor network has been shown to exhibit increased coupling with areas of the autobiographical memory network during traumatic memory retrieval (Kearney, Terpou, et al., 2023). These alterations to neuronal communication may map onto the perception of timeless reexperiencing. In other words, these alterations cause one's perception of time to be disrupted due to lack of connection with their current surroundings, causing the sensations of the past to infiltrate into the present. While Brewin theorized that disrupted traumatic memory processing occurs at the higher-order reflective brain level, future studies should explore the role that the survival brain plays in this process, given that it is the first section to receive these sensations and dictate their respective trajectories in the brain.

Among individuals who experience dissociation, there is a profound disconnection from one's body or surroundings, which can create cracks in the tapestry of one's sense of self (Schiavone et al., 2018). For example, some individuals may think "I am not me anymore" or "I feel like my body has no boundary; I don't know where I begin or end." This unstable sense of self can affect an individual's ability to feel present, and memory retrieval can be difficult since there is an insufficient reference point for an individual to make sense of the multisensory imprint from a past event (Fosha, 2013). Bergouignan, Nyberg, and Ehrsson (2014) identified these difficulties in memory retrieval as mediated by the posterior hippocampus, where memories encoded during experimentally induced out-of-body experiences were linked to reduced activation of the posterior hippocampus. Moreover, a recent study by Bergouignan and colleagues suggested that memories encoded during out-of-body experiences are remembered in the third-person perspective rather than in the first-person—therefore, engaging in spatial reorientation of a memory may be a critical target in a therapeutic setting. These findings indicate that dissociative processes that occur during traumatic events, such as dissociative amnesia and out-of-body experiences, can affect one's perception of their surroundings and, in turn, impair encoding processes. Nevertheless, the sensory traces of these memory imprints often linger in a fragmented and confused manner. Without proper context, these sensations can continue to be immensely triggering alongside the inability to pinpoint why or how they are relevant to the traumatic event.

Mainstream Cognitive Treatments May Benefit from a Sensory-Minded Approach

As discussed above, traumatic memories can have a timeless nature where they are relived as sensory fragments rather than remembered as an integrated memory of the past. This impedes the full integration of traumatic memories across all sections of the brain. If the sensory imprints comprising past traumatic memories prevent the reflective brain from being fully engaged, cognitively oriented treatments may have a suboptimal effect, which may explain why some individuals initially do not respond to these interventions. Given that the threatened brain's locus of control lies with the survival brain, the brain is primarily focused on discerning threat versus safety in the environment rather than reflecting on the present surroundings and applying appropriate context and meaning to traumatic memories. Even if trauma-related beliefs stemming from raw affect, arousal, and sensations evoked from past traumatic memories may be identified, an individual may feel stuck within a threat-dominated state, limiting their capacity to challenge these beliefs. While a Socratic dialogue may be useful in some respects, it cannot achieve its full potential if one has a limited capacity to engage the reflective brain responsible for understanding complex emotions. For many, escaping the grip of disorienting sensations and visceral anguish seems a Houdini-level feat, precluding the capacity to challenge strongly held trauma-related beliefs. Tragically, this reiteration of perceived failure may perpetuate feelings of shame and inadequacy among trauma survivors.

Based on our current understanding of the brain, engaging the reflective brain section would be a critical *final* step for trauma processing, rather than the initial step. The most effective course of action may be to start by reengaging all three sections of the brain through sensory- and arousal-informed approaches in the promotion of dynamic neuronal synchrony. This dynamic synchrony across all brain sections can begin by anchoring in the external and internal worlds (e.g., mindfulness, focused movements) through orienting to safe sensory stimuli. This approach can eventually lay the prerequisite foundation for a reflective brain that feels safe and grounded enough to challenge its own belief systems. Furthermore, engaging the reflective brain consumes precious energy required for the survival brain to be on high alert, detecting any potential threat. Ultimately, *if you feel unsafe, if your survival brain overshadows your conscious experience, if the sense of your body in the present is significantly altered, your ability to challenge your thoughts becomes profoundly diminished.* Without attending to the needs of the whole brain, having the traumatized cortex fully online feels unsafe and may even be impossible. Therefore, orienting the traumatized individual to safety in the external and internal worlds at the onset of treatment may be a gateway for cognitively focused treatments to achieve their full potential (see Bridging to Practice 3 for additional guidance to implement in a therapeutic setting).

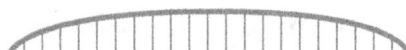

BRIDGING TO PRACTICE 3

Sensory Mindfulness: Nurturing the Connection between the Bodily Self and the Environment

As discussed in the chapter, external sources of sensory information are always accompanied by some form of inner visceral sensations, more commonly referred to as our "gut feelings." These sensations are often processed at a preconscious or subconscious level in the survival brain that lies outside of the individual's awareness. Therefore, an individual may experience a sensation and respond to it before it travels through the upper brain layers to aid with further identification or interpretation. Among traumatized individuals, sustained states of hypervigilance can predispose them to a perpetual feeling that the world is unsafe. Thus, the survival brain would be more likely to experience any sensation, whether pleasant or unpleasant, as a sign of danger and elicit a panic response without any further interpretation in the upper brain layers.

If an individual is unaware of how their body reacts to internal and external sensations and the brain's systematic response to them, they can feel disoriented and unaware of how to manage their inner anguish. This can be difficult for *both* the client and the therapist to navigate because an overwhelming sensory trigger may be an unknown traumatic reminder for the client and thus difficult to process. For example, a beautiful red flower may seem benign, but the visual sensation it evokes may be reminiscent of witnessing a bloody assault due to the same red coloring. Therefore, it is imperative to encourage *sensory mindfulness* by dissecting any unpleasant experience of a client in a nonjudgmental, curious manner, to shed light on these seemingly benign sensations. The therapist can encourage the client to gradually sit and stay with the raw affect, even at first for a few seconds, then 30 seconds, and then up to a minute, using the therapeutic environment as a safe space in which to experience these likely intense visceral sensations. Here, the client and therapist can dissect these triggers, breaking them down into the different sensory components (e.g., visual, auditory, smell, gustatory, tactile, vestibular, proprioceptive, interoceptive) and helping clients map them to their traumatic experiences to piece them together. As the length of time that the client sits with these sensations increases, the client can gain further understanding of the relationship of these sensations to past and present experiences and have better insight into how the raw affect is experienced at lower levels of the brain (see the illustration below).

Sensory Mindfulness: Feel, Locate, Notice, and Reflect

Reflective brain	How does it feel? Where do I feel it? What does it mean? Does it relate to my past?
Emotional learning brain	Is the sensation associated with a positive or negative feeling? Does a past experience come up?
Survival brain	Raw sensations and arousal are reflected as feelings in the body.

Over time, the client may become less reactive and hypo-/hypervigilant to these sensations, allowing these triggering sensations to be transmitted to the upper layers of the brain for deeper processing. The figure above can be used to illustrate this concept to clients, showing how each section of the brain experiences sensations differently. In the survival brain, these sensations are experienced as gut sensations that elicit raw affect, where the body may react to protect itself if they carry a greater intensity. However, if an individual can sit with this affect, it can be transmitted to the limbic emotional brain system to identify the emotional valence of the sensation (e.g., positive or negative) and connect it with past experiences that may come up simultaneously. Eventually, this sensation can reach the cortical reflective brain layer for deeper processing. This brain layer facilitates a more complex understanding of the emotional connection between triggering sensations and a traumatic experience, allowing the individual to become more cognizant of how their body responds. This increased capacity for reflection can give individuals a sense of control and lay a foundation for reframing these sensations. Here, the therapeutic dyad can explore and discuss these sensations with a newfound understanding and reduce their emotional intensity to alleviate the burden of their inner anguish.

Questions to ask your client:

1. Was there an event or experience that happened over the past week that bothered you, but you do not know why?
2. Can you describe the inner bodily sensation that came up during this experience? Where did you feel it in your body? Ask about the feet, stomach, chest, neck, and facial areas. You can use the diagrams in Bridging to Practice 1 to help with this exercise.
3. Can you describe the different sensations in your surroundings during this experience? Ask about visual, auditory, gustatory, tactile, smell, and vestibular sensations.
4. How long did you sit with this sensation?
5. If you feel comfortable, it might be helpful to sit with this sensation for just a bit longer to understand how it is affecting you. Would you be willing to try this at some point?
6. After sitting with this sensation for a bit longer, were there any past experiences that came up? Was the feeling pleasant or unpleasant?
7. Are there any words that come up for you as you sit with this sensation?
8. How do you think these words may relate to the past?
9. How do you think these sensations may relate to the past? Does it relate to feelings of past experiences?

Examples of activities that help to understand inner visceral sensations:

1. Going for a walk with a client, encouraging them to pay attention to their surroundings and pay particular attention to visceral sensations that come up.

2. Using the diagram above, which illustrates how sensory information is carried throughout the three sections of the brain and their role in understanding sensations, as well as the body's response to triggers.

3. 5–4–3–2–1 grounding strategy: Encourage the client to identify five things they can see, four things they can touch, three things they can hear, two things they can smell, and one thing they can taste. While this is a grounding technique, it can also be used to help the client identify sensations that feel *safe* to them. If an individual can sit with these sensations, it can also be used to teach the client how sensory information is transmitted through the brain.

4

The Defense Cascade

HOW SENSORY EXPERIENCE
INFORMS THE LINE OF DEFENSE

The same traumatic experience can lead to strikingly different clinical, neuro-physiological, and neurobiological responses. At one time, 20 or 30 years ago, individuals were often thought to have PTSD only if they exhibited increased physiological and emotional responses, such as an increase in heart rate, when faced with reminders of their trauma. In addition, individuals were often excluded from studies if their heart rate did not increase when they were reminded of their trauma. Around this time, one of us got ready to perform her first brain scans with individuals who were suffering from PTSD. These brain scans used functional magnetic resonance imaging (fMRI) to track blood flow in the brain when individuals recalled traumatic experiences. Brain regions that exhibited increased blood flow were thought to be involved in traumatic memory recall.

The following cases underscore the significance of individual differences in how people subjectively experience and biologically respond to traumatic memories, as related to different defensive responses as discussed in this chapter.

Case Examples: Too Much or Too Little—
A Tale of Two Trauma Responses

The first case involved a husband and wife who were both diagnosed with PTSD, each displaying distinct subjective, psychophysiological, and neurobiological reactions to their traumatic experience (see Lanius, Hopper, & Menon, 2003). The couple survived a severe motor vehicle accident involving over 100 vehicles, multiple fatalities, and severe injuries. During the accident, they were trapped in their car for several minutes and witnessed the tragic death of a child by fire, leaving them feeling helpless and fearing for their lives. They underwent assessments using a heart rate monitor and a brain scan to measure their responses when recalling the traumatic memory of their car accident.

Upon recalling their traumatic experiences while in the brain scanner, the husband exhibited intense anxiety and heightened arousal, accompanied by a 13 beats-per-minute increase in heart rate; he had thoughts focused on escape. The brain scan revealed increased blood flow to various brain regions, including the amygdala in the emotional learning brain section, which was likely related to the husband's increased arousal. In the reflective brain, he also showed activation in visual areas, likely associated with visual flashbacks, as well as frontal regions, related to actively planning how to escape from the car in a flashback during the brain scan.

By stark contrast, the wife described feeling emotionally "numb" and "frozen" while recalling the car accident in the brain scanner. She showed no change in heart rate and exhibited a "shut-down" brain, which showed brain activation only in the visual brain regions likely related to her visual flashbacks during the brain scan. (See Plate 4.1.)

Suzy was another patient who had their brain scanned and showed patterns similar to those of the wife described above. Suzy had suffered from chronic PTSD, and she had been hospitalized for a total of 3 years. Suzy had a severe history of childhood trauma, where she was not only sexually assaulted by several relatives but also repeatedly shamed, ridiculed, and beaten by her mother. Indeed, her mother told her that she wished she had not been born. Suzy described that she survived her childhood by hiding and staying still, akin to a freezing response. Prior to having her brain scan, Suzy was asked to provide a narrative of her traumatic experiences, which was then read back to her while she was in the scanner. When Suzy recalled one of her childhood traumas, she felt like she was reliving the past. She eloquently described how she felt disconnected from her body and felt "frozen" and unable to move, a response that allowed her to survive her childhood because it prevented her from being seen and heard. To our great surprise, Suzy's heart rate decreased while she was recalling her traumatic childhood memory while having her brain scanned. In addition, her brain seemed to shut down—very little activation was observed throughout her brain. Suzy's brain scan marked the beginning of a paradigm shift in the study of PTSD. From then on, it became clear that individuals could have both hyperarousal and/or blunted arousal responses to recalling their trauma. It was therefore critical to simultaneously monitor individuals' clinical, neurophysiological, and/or biological responses and to pay close attention to the individual's subjective report of their suffering.

Overview of the ANS

The ANS is a highly evolutionarily conserved system that is designed to help individuals respond to stress in a timely, flexible manner. It plays a crucial role in maintaining the body's homeostasis, helping to balance our natural physiological processes throughout the body. This includes the regulation of blood pressure, digestion, urinary retention, and internal body temperature (McCorry, 2007). The ANS has two branches, which have opposing yet complementary functions: the sympathetic nervous system, characterized by the fight-or-flight response, and the parasympathetic nervous system, which initiates restorative processes (Ondicova & Mravec, 2010; Valenza, Ciò, Toschi, & Barbieri, 2024). Notably, the ANS functions without conscious or voluntary control.

The sympathetic nervous system is activated when the body experiences any form of stressor. In the body, stress is signaled through sensations from the external and internal worlds, which are then directed to the survival brain. Interoceptive sensations are transmitted through somatosensory pathways and cranial nerve X, the vagus nerve, and converge at the brainstem to intersect signals from the brain and body (McCorry, 2007). This incoming sensory information is further signaled from the survival brain to the hypothalamus, a structure in the emotional learning brain, to activate the sympathetic nervous system and facilitate cortisol release to initiate the body's fight-or-flight response (Adler & Geenen, 2005; Ondicova & Mravec, 2010; Valenza et al., 2024). This is the body's primal response to threat in preparation for fighting or fleeing from a predator, characterized by increased heart rate, shortness of breath, and increased adrenaline. Moreover, the sympathetic nervous system is mediated by acetylcholine and norepinephrine, neurotransmitters produced in the brainstem regions, such as the locus coeruleus, which increase blood flow to critical organs in the body, including the heart, muscles, and the brain itself (Weihe et al., 2005).

When a calm state is considered adaptive, such as in conditions of safety, the parasympathetic nervous system is engaged to modulate activities associated with "rest" and digestion (McCorry, 2007).

Escapable versus Inescapable Stress: Acute versus Chronic

After trauma, there is long-term disruption to the ANS due in part to adaptations associated with prolonged stress. Hans Selye (1950) was one of the first scientists to describe the body's biological stress response as a phasic process, starting with the alarm reaction phase, then entering the resistance phase, and finally arriving at the exhaustion phase:

- The alarm reaction phase is the body's initial response to stress and is analogous to the body's fight-or-flight response.

• In the resistance stage, the body attempts to repair itself after the initial shock of stress, eliciting different reactions depending on whether the stressor is acute (lasting for a short period) or chronic (persisting and/or inescapable). If the stressor is acute and has dissipated, the physiological state of the body attempts to return to prestress levels (e.g., decreased heart rate, slower breathing). However, if the stressor is chronic, the body never receives a concrete signal to restore levels of normal functioning and will continue secretion of stress hormones that sustain physiological arousal within the body. This results in further chronic disruptions, such as bowel issues, headaches, and irritability.

• This state of prolonged stress eventually instigates the final exhaustion phase, where chronic stress depletes the body's physical, emotional, and mental resources meant to cope with stress. This exhaustion phase can give rise to chronic medical and autoimmune conditions, where the body cannot fully recover after stress (Maté, 2011; Maté & Maté, 2022; McEwen, 2013; Nakazawa, 2015, 2021). Unsurprisingly, this final stage substantially impacts an individual's quality of life due to persistent fatigue, poor cardiovascular health, and decreased stress tolerance.

Defense Cascade Model of the Stress Response

The defense cascade model builds upon Selye's (1950) stress model by further describing how organisms respond to various types of threat (Kozlowska et al., 2015; Lanius et al., 2017; Schauer & Elbert, 2010). It proposes that defensive responses occur on a continuum and are mediated by brain pathways originating in the survival and emotional learning brains, including the hypothalamus and the amygdala in the emotional learning brain, as well as the periaqueductal gray and the presympathetic and vagal nuclei deep in the survival brain. While this model is based on animal literature and has not yet been explicitly examined in humans, several authors have pointed to key similarities between defensive mechanisms in humans and defensive responses in other animals (Kozlowska et al., 2015; Lanius et al., 2017; Schauer & Elbert, 2010).

We focus our discussion on the defense cascade model with reference to two types of threat: escapable threat and inescapable threat. As the term implies, *escapable threat* involves a stressor where escape is possible, such as being able to take cover from a hurricane or managing to fight off an assailant during an assault. By contrast, inescapable threat involves a stressor that one cannot evade, as is evident during chronic childhood abuse or prolonged episodes of torture. Both types of threat initiate distinct brain pathways that elicit different biological responses, as described in the cases above. Below we describe each stage of the defense cascade model in the context of both escapable and inescapable threat. The stages include the orienting freeze, fight-or-flight, freezing/tonic immobility, and emotional

TABLE 4.1. The Autonomic Nervous System and Stages of the Defense Cascade Model, Compared

	Fight or flight	Tonic immobility/freezing	Emotional shutdown
Pupils	Dilated	Dilated	Constricted
Pain threshold	Decreased	Increased	Increased
Voice production	Available	Restricted, jaws clasped	Absent
Body temperature	Increased	Cold at extremities	Coldest
Digestion	Decreased	Decreased	Bowels released
Breathing, heart rate	Increased	Increased	Low
Muscle tone	Increased	Most tense	Flaccid

shutdown (see Table 4.1). As we see, the fight-or-flight stage is dominated by the sympathetic nervous system, the freezing/tonic immobility stage by both branches of the ANS, and the emotional shutdown stage by the parasympathetic nervous system.

Orienting Freeze

When a predator or threat is first detected, the superior colliculus and the periaqueductal gray in the survival brain receive sensory information from the external surroundings and from within the body, swiftly eliciting an orienting "freeze" response. This response can also be considered the "STOP, LOOK, LISTEN" response, as it serves to orient the organism as to its location and postural position in space in relation to the threat. In this context, the superior colliculus acts as a "radar" in terms of monitoring an organism's disposition and, if a potentially emotionally relevant or threatening stimulus is detected, sends signals to coordinate a defensive response. The periaqueductal gray initiates a small dip in arousal via its connections to brainstem autonomic centers as the organism responds to the threat (Corrigan, Fisher, & Nutt, 2011; Corrigan & Grand, 2013; Kozlowska et al., 2015; Lanius et al., 2017; Schauer & Elbert, 2010).

Fight-or-Flight

The most adaptive outcome of the defense cascade is when one has the capacity to flee from the threat. This outcome, mediated by the lateral portion of the periaqueductal gray, makes use of the sympathetic nervous system response and its concomitant surge of stress hormones (e.g., adrenaline). If the organism is not capable of fleeing from the threat, the next most adaptive response is to fight the threat or predator. Here, more adrenaline is released to provide the organism with even more fuel to actively defend itself and overcome the threat.

Physiologically, the body's fight-or-flight response is characterized by increased heart rate, shallow breathing, and dilated pupils in preparation for the organism to fight or flee from the predator. Moreover, blood vessels and skeletal muscles constrict, increasing blood pressure and muscle tone. Urination is stimulated through contraction of the bladder sphincter while digestive processes, such as gastric fluid secretion and peristalsis, are inhibited. Additionally, the presence of acute stress can increase body temperature and induce psychogenic fevers, where core body temperature can run up to 105° F (41° C) compared to 98.6° F (37° C) (Oka, 2015; Oka & Oka, 2012).

An integral component of sympathetic nervous system activation is the endogenous cannabinoid system, which mediates release of pain-relieving neurotransmitters called endocannabinoids. Endocannabinoid signaling occurs at the level of the dorsal-lateral periaqueductal gray and acts as an analgesic during the fight-or-flight response, subsequently reducing the availability of cannabinoid receptors. In turn, endocannabinoid secretion induces hyperactivity of the amygdala in the emotional learning brain and perpetuates hyperarousal and hypervigilance symptoms in the face of a traumatic event, where individuals may be hypersensitive to their surroundings (Lanius et al., 2018).

Traumatized individuals often become trapped in a state of reliving, perpetuated through ongoing fight-or-flight defensive responses. When the horrifying past feels like the present and threat seems forever imminent, it is no wonder that traumatized individuals appear to be combative and uncooperative. These behaviors should be clinically identified through the lens of the body's primal urge to defend itself, an urge evoked subconsciously at the level of the survival brain. It is also paramount for observers and clinicians to view these behavioral responses as subconsciously evoked rather than as volitionally manipulative or malicious in nature, as is representative of a primary conduct disorder. Otherwise, one risks labeling traumatized individuals as "bad" or "noncompliant," which can have devastating consequences, as we illustrate in the case of Johnny, "The Defiant Child." While this is not an excuse for damaging behaviors, this explanation provides a neuroscientifically guided framework to emphasize why it is crucial to target the behaviors at their survival brain roots. Without the reflective brain fully online, higher-level cognitive interventions, which require a capacity for reflection that is not yet accessible, can be energy depleting and defeating for the client. This is consistent with neuroscientific literature, which has shown that the ventromedial prefrontal cortex, responsible for attentional processing, voluntary actions, and threat appraisal, is suboptimally engaged in traumatized individuals. In the end, this leaves the survival brain with the primary locus of control (Hansel & von Kanel, 2008; Harricharan et al., 2021; Kearney & Lanius, 2022).

CASE EXAMPLE: Johnny, "The Defiant Child"

Johnny is a 15-year-old teenager, a middle child between an older sister and a younger brother. As a child, Johnny was vibrant and curious; he loved to spend countless hours in the garden crafting beautiful sandcastles with his siblings. To Johnny's parents, he was very loving and affectionate. He excelled at school, regularly impressing his teachers with his academic and artistic talents. After an event at age 12, however, that all changed.

Johnny tragically witnessed the death of his younger brother in a car accident. After this horrifying and shocking event, Johnny's way of being in the world changed abruptly. He appeared perpetually angry and hostile, regularly instigating and engaging in fights at home and at school. His family and his peers started to fear him. Johnny's schoolwork began to suffer as he lost interest in all the academic and artistic pursuits that he previously enjoyed. Both his parents and his teachers became increasingly frustrated by Johnny's "bad" and "defiant" behavior. Johnny became more and more isolated at school and increasingly began to be labeled as an "oppositionally defiant" teenager. His behavior escalated over the next 2 years, and he was almost expelled for aggressive behavior.

Fortunately, Johnny's parents found a therapist for Johnny when he was 14 years old. While getting to know Johnny, his therapist pieced together the correspondence of his having witnessed the tragic death of his brother with the onset of his challenging behaviors and simmering anger. The therapist realized that Johnny felt trapped in a state of reliving the memory of his brother's accident, which caused chronic fight responses manifesting as aggressive behavior. His therapist met with his parents and his teachers to help them make sense of Johnny's "outrageous" behaviors, initially emphasizing cognitive strategies that challenged his aggressive thoughts and behaviors. However, Johnny was unable to apply or benefit from these strategies, likely due to suboptimal access to his prefrontal cortex, which is the critical neural target for cognitive-behavioral approaches. His therapist realized that she needed to use an alternative approach to get through to Johnny. She formulated an integrative trauma-focused approach targeting sensorimotor arousal regulation in conjunction with training brain wave activity through neurofeedback. Over the next several months, he became less aggressive and less easily startled, and he was able to calm down within minutes instead of hours. His focus also improved, which returned Johnny to routine engagement in his academic and artistic activities. Due to his restored concentration and newfound capacity for reflection, his therapist was able to utilize those same cognitive-behavioral approaches to help Johnny form a narrative of his brother's accident, make meaning of the horrific event, and process his grief. Johnny's return to inner peace allowed him to enjoy comfort and joy with his family once again.

Freezing/Tonic Immobility (Feigned Death)

When danger is deemed inescapable, progressed past the point of any potential for survival, a state of freezing/tonic immobility can ensue. Tonic immobility is an involuntary self-preservation state characterized by the sudden onset of muscle rigidity to produce a physically immobile state. This involuntary muscle rigidity is a way for the threatened individual to feign death in an attempt to prevent further attack from the predator. Autonomically, the "traditional" view is that the sympathetic and parasympathetic branches work to counterbalance each other—however, it is now thought that the two branches can be coactivated, or activated simultaneously. This has been observed during the tonic immobility response as heart rate becomes controlled by both the sympathetic and parasympathetic branches of the ANS. In animal research on tonic immobility, the sympathetic nervous system has been shown to remain activated to maintain an increased heart rate and a readiness of large muscle groups to act while the parasympathetic nervous system begins to initiate a "parasympathetic brake" on the heart to slow it down as a way to evade the predator—this brake can be quickly removed to allow the body to swiftly flee to safety if given the opportunity (Alm, 2004; Skora, Livermore, & Roelofs, 2022). Studies have also shown that the tonic immobility state is accompanied by a decrease in heart rate variability and reduction in body sway (Norte et al., 2019; Volchan et al., 2011).

Humans who enter this state describe feeling "encased in cement." The characteristic muscle rigidity can be paralyzing to a point of immobility in all or some parts of the body, including limbs, the intercostal breathing muscles, and/or the eye muscles involved in visual tracking. Specifically, stiffness in the intercostal breathing muscles can lead to shallow breathing, making it difficult to take a full, deep breath. In addition, an inability to move the eye muscles can result in a "frozen" gaze, an often terrifying experience that leads the individual to feel like they are a "deer caught in headlights," unable to defend themselves or others.

From a clinical perspective, the inability to act may evoke feelings of defectiveness or weakness, which can precipitate feelings of guilt and shame (Lloyd et al., 2019). Even though freezing/tonic immobility serves as an adaptive defensive response under conditions of inescapable threat, posttraumatic reengagement of this type of defensive responding comes at a cost. In the aftermath of repeated trauma, chronic tonic immobility/freezing can rob an individual of their agency and control over their own actions, leaving them to feel trapped in their bodies, misunderstood and invisible to the world.

CASE EXAMPLE: Overcoming Tonic Immobility/Freezing Using Deep Pressure

A 52-year-old man named Jimmy has a long-standing history of dissociation, particularly freezing/tonic immobility responses to certain events or stimuli several times a day. The frequency and severity of his defensive responses require him to have a service dog, Skip, with him at all times. In particular, Jimmy reacts with a frozen, immobilized posture when he is directly asked a question, due to a pervasive fear of giving the "wrong answer." This very real fear dates back to his childhood, where his mother would severely and repeatedly punish him whenever he seemed to say the "wrong" thing.

While Jimmy was initially interactive with his new therapist, his demeanor shifted suddenly when he was asked to share his homework assignment from the previous session. He became still and motionless, holding a frozen and expressionless gaze that looked right through the therapist. Jimmy maintained this stunned state for an extended time, unable to vocalize his thoughts. Even though the therapist felt somewhat uneasy, she knew that Jimmy was having a freezing/tonic immobility response that had routinely helped him to feel hidden and invisible so as to not get hurt by his threatening mother throughout his childhood. Instinctively, Skip could tell that Jimmy was frozen within the therapy session and intentionally placed his body weight on Jimmy's lap to help bring him out of this state. After about 5 minutes of sustained deep pressure from Skip, Jimmy started to feel safe enough to begin reorienting to the present.

The therapist and Jimmy conducted a behavioral analysis of the experience, realizing the sensation of deep pressure elicits a grounding effect that can help him reemerge from the freezing/tonic immobility state. The therapist inquired whether he would be open to intermittent use of a weighted vest or belt to mimic the dog's pressure in order to decrease the intensity and frequency of future freezing episodes.

The state of freezing/tonic immobility is an evolutionarily conserved state that is readily reversible if the threat dissipates, where the organism can quickly revert to fleeing the threat and finding safety. However, among individuals who experience chronic and/or severe traumatization (e.g., repeated abuse, chronic neglect, childhood sexual abuse, and/or prolonged torture), the predator frequently does not lose interest in predation and the individual transitions into the next phase of the stress response.

Emotional Shutdown

If all previous stages of the defense cascade, including the freezing/tonic immobility phase, have been exhausted and the threat remains inescapable, emotional shutdown ensues. Emotional shutdown is mediated by the ventrolateral aspect of the periaqueductal gray, which serves to inhibit motorically active fight-or-flight defensive responses. Here, the organism shows physiological responses consistent with marked parasympathetic overdrive through activation of nuclei in the medulla oblongata, the lowest part of the survival brain. These nuclei include the vagal and parabrachial sensory nuclei as well as the reticular activating system, a survival brain structure key in modulating arousal and muscle tone. Here, the solitary nuclei in the medulla receive incoming signals from the cardiovascular and respiratory systems in the body and translate this to the medulla oblongata and vagus nerve to modify parasympathetic activity (Breit, Kupferberg, Rogler, & Hasler, 2018; Jaradeh & Prieto, 2003). During parasympathetic activation, the heart rate decreases and blood vessels dilate, thereby decreasing blood pressure, which may even cause individuals to faint. Moreover, muscle tone turns flaccid to initiate a transient paralysis, making the body unable to generate movement (Alboni & Alboni, 2014). Flaccidity of muscles can carry over to disrupt the bladder and anal sphincters, which can lead to involuntary urination and defecation, which can be incredibly dehumanizing in the posttraumatic condition.

From a neurochemical perspective, the emotional shutdown response is theorized to be mediated by the endogenous opioid system, specifically the kappa and mu opioid systems. Chronic, inescapable stress activates kappa opioid receptors, which can precipitate negative alterations in mood (e.g., dysphoria) and elicit dissociative symptomatology (e.g., depersonalization and derealization symptoms— see below; Addy, Garcia-Romeu, Metzger, & Wade, 2015). This can be an avenue for chronic feelings of helplessness, demotivation, and depression that are frequently observed in the aftermath of repeated traumatization (Lanius et al., 2018). The kappa opioid system (dynorphin) has also been shown to cause disruptions in consciousness, facilitating significant alterations in the processing of external sensory stimuli and in the perception of inner bodily states, forming the core of dissociation: a psychological, emotional, and sensorial escape when no physical escape is possible (Putnam, 1989). Alternatively, activation of mu opioid receptors can appear as reduced responsiveness to pain, which is a survival strategy invoked to detach from the writhing agony associated with torture, abuse, and neglect. In actuality, traumatized individuals have been shown to have a higher pain threshold when exposed to pain generated from intense heat (Geuze et al., 2007). This may also explain why soldiers in the battlefield may not show a pain response until hours after they were injured in combat (Pitman, van der Kolk, Orr, & Greenberg, 1990).

Importantly, this shutdown response is thought to be associated with *thalamocortical sensory deafferentation*, a disruption in the neural pathways connecting the thalamus and the cortex. The thalamus, a key relay station in the emotional learning brain for the transmission of internal and external sensory stimuli to the cortex, is a place where our awareness and ability to contextualize sensory input coincide. Thalamocortical deafferentation obstructs the normal pathways from the thalamus to the cortex, altering neuronal firing rates and rendering them "out of sync" and suboptimally communicative. Logically, these brain structures need to be firing "in sync" to translate sensory information effectively to higher brain structures critical for everyday functions, such as decision making, language, agency, and emotion regulation. Severing this pathway brilliantly allows the traumatized individual to detach from torturous visceral physical and emotional pain experienced within the body during traumatic events.

In the long term, unfortunately, the lack of communication to the higher levels of the brain about the internal state of the body and the environment may lead to a profound detachment from the body that manifests as "I don't feel, and everything around me feels unreal—life is not really happening." These experiences are known as dissociative phenomena, where depersonalization ("I feel detached from my body") and derealization ("Everything around me feels unreal!") are involuntary coping mechanisms to soothe the inescapable pain. In this state, emerging evidence shows an interruption in the formation of explicit memories (Bergouignan et al., 2014, 2022; Kozlowska et al., 2015; Lanius et al., 2017; Schauer & Elbert, 2010), thereby disrupting normal memory formation. This leads to involuntary and vivid reliving of the trauma in place of voluntarily remembering it as a past occurrence. The traumatized individual is frequently hijacked by sensations and defensive motor responses while reexperiencing the trauma without context or awareness of the present (Brewin, 2014; Brewin et al., 1996; Kearney, Terpou, et al., 2023; van der Kolk & Fisler, 1995).

If this emotional shutdown state of feeling emotionally dead to the world becomes chronic, it can initiate a state of "learned helplessness," a chronic state of depression as is frequently observed in the aftermath of trauma. In learned helplessness, an individual may become unable or unwilling to face subsequent stressful situations, even if they are escapable, due to the initial experience of being unable to escape. This was first observed in dogs by Overmier and Seligman (1967). In one experimental condition, they exposed a dog to an electric shock stimulus in a shuttle box where the dog was able to run frantically to escape the box and successfully evade the shock with increasing efficacy as the number of trials increased. However, in another condition, a dog was exposed to an electric shock stimulus in the same shuttle box but was prevented from escaping by being placed in a Pavlovian hammock. While this dog ran frantically for 30 seconds, it eventually stopped moving, laid down, and quietly cried. Even when escape became possible in subsequent trials, the dog still could not escape, presumably because it had learned it lacked control over its own self-preservation in this situation. Although feeling detached from one's own body and the environment can be a reprieve during inescapable agonizing pain, it can perpetuate a state of "emotional anesthesia" and habitual helplessness, thereby depriving an individual of feeling alive and being an active agent in the world (Kozlowska et al., 2015; Lanius et al., 2017; Schauer & Elbert, 2010; Terpou, Densmore, et al., 2019).

Individuals who are prone to experiencing sustained periods of "emotional anesthesia" may require engagement in extreme sensory-seeking behaviors, including reckless sports, promiscuous sexual behaviors, drug use, and aggression in order to feel alive (Briere, 1992, 2019). Traumatized individuals frequently report being able to overcome emotional stupor only through seeking reckless behaviors that involve extreme sensory and affective (e.g., fear) stimulation. Critically, these intense inputs may be required to overcome the blockage between the thalamus and the cortex, thereby initiating sensory integration and facilitating a level of vigor required to feel a semblance of life. Only through extreme measures can one seem to feel and thereby connect with oneself, others, and the world at large.

Although there is no direct evidence in humans that the likelihood of survival increases in relation to the onset of dissociative or shutdown responses, animal research indicates that these responses are induced by cues that indicate imminent threat, such as mechanical restraint, pointing toward their role in enhancing survival (Gallup & Rager, 1996). Accordingly, future work in humans should examine specifically whether chances of survival increase and/or level of threat decreases in association with tonic immobility or emotional shutdown. Notably, bodily reactions to threat consistent with freezing/tonic immobility have been reported among healthy individuals (Volchan et al., 2017). In particular, when they were shown a threatening image indicating little chance of escape (gun pointing at them), they exhibited reduced body sway and slowed heart rate indicative of tonic immobility. By contrast, pictures consistent with an increased chance of escape (gun pointing away from them) elicited increased body sway, which may suggest preparation for active escape or flight as depicted in the earlier phase of the defense cascade model (Volchan et al., 2017). On balance, the findings reviewed here suggest strongly that the defense cascade model can be applied to humans.

CASE EXAMPLE: How Compassionate Touch Links with Negative Self-Image—A Case of Emotional Shutdown

A young woman named Maya, diagnosed with complex PTSD, borderline personality disorder, and dissociative identity disorder, was intrigued by a flyer advertising research on tactile processing in PTSD: "I've felt like an alien all of my life. I had no idea that I wasn't the only one like this—that my hatred of touch and wearing certain fabrics could be part of my PTSD." During an in-depth psychological assessment, Maya shared her story of severe childhood physical, emotional, and sexual abuse coinciding with poverty and sporadic homelessness. Touch had never been a positive force in her life. Negative experiences with abuse and rape and rejection had resulted in a deep discomfort with interpersonal touch and severe difficulty maintaining romantic relationships. However, her interest in helping others understand their own discomfort with touch motivated her enough to endure an fMRI scan while an experimenter held her hand and presented her with visual displays of personalized neutral, negative, and positive words.

During the neutral word presentation, the experimenter noticed that Maya's hand was limp and cold, indicative of an emotional shutdown response. However, her disposition starkly shifted when her negative words were displayed: "abandoned," "dirty," "broken." The experimenter felt her hand become warm as it squeezed back tightly, seeming to hold on for dear life. At the end of the negative words trial, she reported her answers to questions about how she was feeling in a high-pitched, child-like voice, suggesting a dissociative state shift into her child state characterized by strong fight-or-flight responses. Next came her positive words: "resilient," "strong." Her hand returned to feeling cold and lifeless, similar to the initial emotional shutdown state, and her vocal tone returned to sounding soft and defeated. During the postexperiment debrief, the experimenter asked her how she experienced the sensation of touch during the positive and negative word presentations: "The positive words? It felt uncomfortable, I felt afraid—I felt as if I would contaminate you somehow. The negative words, I can't seem to remember at all." The strongly negative words not only changed how Maya felt emotionally; she experienced a dissociative reenactment of the terrified child state held deep inside, frantically desperate to be held.

CASE EXAMPLE: Linking Emotional Shutdown with the Past— Emerging from the Shadows

Joy is a 50-year-old woman with an extensive history of childhood abuse. Growing up, she felt safe with no one, with the exception of an aunt whom she saw only once a year. Joy struggled with emotional shutdown responses for many years, which manifested as persistent, perpetual dissociation, chronic fatigue, and a general "flatness" to her emotional world. However, her body intuitively combatted these shutdown responses by developing a habit of doing 300–500 push-ups per day. Joy's push-up routine likely started instinctively as an extreme sensation-seeking pattern to reach the threshold required for adequate activation of her sympathetic nervous system in compensation for the parasympathetic overdrive associated with her shutdown states.

Joy was unfortunately injured during a workplace accident one day, and she suffered a shoulder injury that prevented her from engaging in her regular push-ups. After this incident, Joy's shutdown responses were exacerbated. She collapsed into a fetal position when faced with a reminder of her past traumatic experiences, causing her muscles to turn limp, her heart rate and blood pressure to decrease significantly, and her memory to go blank for minutes to hours. She was seen by various medical practitioners who were puzzled by what was happening. Eventually, Joy was referred to a psychiatrist who became aware that Joy was experiencing emotional shutdown responses associated with a chronic history of inescapable childhood trauma. During therapy, Joy realized that these shutdown responses were linked to her childhood traumatic experiences. This offered her great relief since she could now identify the reason her body had been reacting the way it was throughout her life.

Joy worked with her therapist to activate her sympathetic nervous system through exercises that did not compromise her shoulder injury. Joy became very adept at rapidly cycling on a stationary bike. Over time, these compensatory strategies helped to stabilize her ANS by way of a more adaptive balance of sympathetic and parasympathetic nervous system activity, leading to a significant reduction in the severity and frequency of her emotional shutdown responses. The cycling replaced the push-ups needed to activate her sympathetic nervous system and overcome her severe emotional shutdown states, leading to greater mental clarity and increased readiness to process her previous traumatic experiences.

Window of Tolerance Model through the Lens of Inescapable versus Escapable Threat

The notion that traumatic experiences alter ANS functioning translates clinically to Daniel J. Siegel's (1999) window of tolerance model of autonomic arousal. This model describes a continuum of arousal states from parasympathetically dominated hypoarousal to sympathetically driven hyperarousal. The optimal zone, or the "window of tolerance," is characterized by an emotionally regulated state that promotes groundedness, flexibility, curiosity, and capacity to tolerate life's stressors. If the window becomes eclipsed, one can enter a state associated with hyperarousal, analogous to the sympathetic fight-or-flight response, or hypoarousal, analogous to the parasympathetically driven emotional shutdown response (Corrigan et al., 2011; d'Andrea et al., 2013). During a freezing/tonic immobility state, an individual can give the impression of being hypoaroused due to their stunned and frozen facial expressions—however, it is more analogous to a hyperarousal state given that an individual still shows increased heart rate, muscle rigidity, and muscular and physiological preparation to initiate fight-or-flight defensive responses if conditions permit (Corrigan et al., 2011). There are also transitional states just outside the window of tolerance, known as fluid zones (Warner, Finn, Westcott, Cook, & Blaustein, 2020), where arousal is on the edge of hyper-/hypoarousal but the individual can still be reached and engaged. This is where therapeutic change is most optimally achieved (see Plate 4.2; see also Bridging to Practice 4 for guidance for how to implement this strategy in therapeutic settings).

A Secure Base Unveiling a Window for Discovery: The Defense Cascade and Beyond

The ANS is the brain and body's thermostat, as it maintains balanced arousal in response to the happenings of inner and outer sensory and emotional life. Just like a thermostat, the brain and body are constantly, but subconsciously, working to maintain an optimal steady state that creates an inner balance of bodily functions (i.e., hormonal balance, blood sugar, immune responses). This steady state can be adapted depending on situational stressors that exist within the external and internal environment, as we have seen.

Starting in utero, mothers begin to establish subliminal bidirectional dynamic communication with their fetus. The fetus remains encapsulated in a safe, soothing environment rich with somatosensory and vestibular input from the womb and movements of the mother. This bidirectional communication in a context of safety fosters the development of basic survival-oriented capacities known as *allostasis*, or the body's ability to respond to stress and regain its desired steady state (McEwen, 2013; Sterling, 2012). It is within this steady, balanced state that we are able to develop and fully connect to our sense of self, others, and the world.

As self-representations begin to take shape in the context of the mother–child attachment relationship, Ciaunica, Safron, and Delafield-Butt (2021) postulated that there are multiple pathways to update self-representations—for example, perceptual inference and active inference. *Perceptual inference* (Friston, 2010) involves updating one's representation based on sensory inputs perceived by the body. For instance, if a child experiences emotional distress, they may hear the frequency of the mother's voice while she is rocking, hugging, and soothing them as they cope with their sadness and distress. This forms a secure base that the young child becomes reliant upon for their first few years to cope with autonomic dysregulation—when their steady state is compromised. In *active inference* (Brown, Adams, Parees, Edwards, & Friston, 2013; Friston, FitzGerald, Rigoli, Schwartenbeck, & Pezzulo, 2017), the child invokes an action that actively seeks the care of their mother to fulfill natural physiological needs in pursuit of a steady state. Among children with a secure base, the child can cry and approach their mother to be soothed and the mother predictably responds with care, reinforcing an unconditionally loving relationship. However, among individuals who lack a secure base, distress may have been met with negative emotion or ignored by their caregiver. Here, the child may initiate an abrupt action to elicit the attention of their caregiver, such as throwing something in the mother's face or hitting the mother. An outside observer could interpret this behavior as "bad" or "oppositionally defiant"—however, this is a desperate attachment response evoked by the child as a plea to their caregiver on whom they depend for survival.

In our most vulnerable developmental years, negative attention is better than no attention. Indeed, developmental costs associated with maternal withdrawal have been shown to be the strongest predictor of the later development of depression, suicidality, self-harm, dissociation, eating disturbances, and borderline personality disorder (Khoury, Pechtel, Andersen, Teicher, & Lyons-Ruth, 2019; Lyons-Ruth & Yarger, 2022). If the child continues to be ignored despite their desperate pleas for connection, the child eventually submits and enters a state of emotional anesthesia, where a sense of agency is lost, and feelings of chronic learned helplessness ensue into adulthood. Importantly, learned helplessness refers to chronic situations of neglect where "adequate" caregiver responses are not present at least 30% of the time (Bretherton, 1992; Hesse & Main, 2000; Tronick & Beeghly, 2011).

The Wheel of Discovery: Seeking Safety or Defense in the Quest to Thrive

A secure base is a compass that guides discovery within and beyond representations of the self. It also promotes a wide window of tolerance, where arousal can fluctuate substantially in the face of a variety of situational demands without entering hyper- or hypoaroused states. A wide window of tolerance fosters a felt sense of safety that permits a curiosity-based seeking of novelty, pleasure, and positive reward. Panksepp defined the SEEKING disposition as the drive underlying exploration and approach behaviors that sustain goal-directed activities and evoke feelings of anticipation and excitement, ultimately influencing reward-based learning (Alcaro & Panksepp, 2011). When a threat is posed, the biological defense cascade response is initiated as described above—however, with a secure base, a person can dynamically adapt to situations without entering autonomic dysregulation and thrive despite challenges or setbacks. This is depicted on the left in Plate 4.3, where a child's secure base forms the hub of a wheel advancing on an ever-changing terrain.

Finding Synchrony and Rhythm with Others: The Polarity between Play and Recklessness

According to Panksepp (2004), CARE or nurturance is another primal form of SEEKING. CARE starts in the womb through co-embodiment of the child and the parent. In fact, being carried by another human being in the womb may be one of the only common threads among all humans. After birth, humans, like many other species, continue to need the CARE of other beings to survive and reproduce. Furthermore, Panksepp postulated that CARE is the underlying system for empathy. Without CARE, relations with our world through our senses are disrupted. For example, recent studies (Maier, Heinen-Ludwig, Gunturkun, Hurlemann, & Scheele, 2020) have shown that children who experienced maltreatment experience higher sensitivity to touch and a decrease in reactivity to affective touch as adults. As our senses shape our perceptions, our agency and interaction with others may be hampered in the face of adversity. Studies have also shown that the parent's attachment style is one of the greatest predictors of their child's attachment style as an adult (van IJzendoorn, 1995). Childhood maltreatment experienced by women had a positive linear relationship with the probability of reporting interpersonal violence—for men, childhood physical abuse predicted the same (Shields, Tonmyr, Hovdestad, Gonzalez, & MacMillan, 2020).

When lacking a secure base, a narrow window of tolerance perpetuates extreme oscillations in arousal states, causing the individual to become stuck in defensive states (Siegel, 1999). Without a sturdy centralized hub, the wheel cannot adapt to the ever-changing terrain and instead becomes stuck, wobbly, or veers off course. As the individual frequently feels unsure and unsafe, they are unable to seek creative or social outlets and instead seek relief from their discomfort. In these cases, seeking can predominantly become directed toward negatively valenced experiences or other "drugs" of choice, such as toxic relationships, addictions, or recklessness, that can reach extremely high sensory thresholds and offer rushes of adrenaline (Maté, 2010; Robinson & Berridge, 2008). Here, the body naturally seeks extreme sensory experiences as fuel to drive the wheel forward and find reprieve from these chronic defensive states (Felitti et al., 1998).

Conversely, if a child is leaping from a secure base, SEEKING will underlie increased interactions with the environment and others in the form of PLAY. PLAY is a similarly innate drive that underlies prosocial interactions and starts before the child is 1 year old (some authors postulate 4–6 weeks) in the form of a social smile. Throughout the child's development, PLAY is inextricably linked with sensorimotor development, which is critical for sensory processing throughout all sections of the brain and can take various forms, such as roughhousing, tag, hide-and-seek, construction, and dramatic pretend play (Feldman, 2007; Piaget, 1962; Trevarthen & Aitken, 2001). This sets the brain up to optimally regulate both arousal and emotional states and allows children to flexibly adapt and attune to their environment. Here, they can feel safe enough to explore and connect with others but also accurately detect threat and seek safety with a caregiver (Zanetti, Powell, Cooper, & Hoffman, 2011).

CASE EXAMPLE: Lola—Scaffolding an Insecure Base

Lola is a vivacious 6-year-old girl who has been in the foster care system since early in her infancy. Her mother suffered domestic violence throughout her pregnancy and left Lola's father after her birth. However, her mother became involved in another abusive relationship shortly thereafter and began using heroin with her new partner. This led to significant physical and emotional neglect of Lola, as well as physical abuse from her mother and her mother's new partner, particularly when they struggled with withdrawal symptoms. Lola was removed from her mother by child protective services at the age of 8 months and placed in the foster care system. Having been torn from her main attachment figure in addition to experiencing significant trauma and stress, Lola was difficult to soothe and labeled as "hyperactive," rendering her unmanageable for many foster parents. As a result, she was shuffled from home to home for the first 4 years of her life. At the age of 4, Lola finally landed with a foster family that had experience with two other traumatized foster children and planned to adopt her.

For those first 4 years, terror, chaos, and unpredictability were all that Lola knew, which scaffolded her internal landscape. Her body and brain had developed to be on constant alert, and she felt confused and uncomfortable in relationally and environmentally safe situations. Lola had significant difficulties with self-regulation, or the ability to soothe herself, because she had never been co-regulated by an attuned adult in her formative months and years. This manifested as an inability to sit and pay attention at school, deal with frustrations with peers on the playground, stay asleep at night, or feel connected and trusting of her new caregivers. In addition, Lola needed to exert control over her external environment and other people to deal with the chaos and unpredictability of her internal world. When anything unexpected happened, such as a change to her routine, she fell apart; emotional meltdowns and physical aggression were daily occurrences. Lola's disconnection from the safety of her own body, stemming from the absence of attuned sensory experiences with a caregiver since birth, resulted in a sense of disconnect from everyone and everything around her. She was frequently in trouble at school, engendering a continual sense of failure.

Lola began occupational therapy after her teachers noticed that she experienced "sensory processing challenges," such as hypersensitivities to noise, touch, and smell. In a frantic attempt to re-create familiar sensations of terror, she also sought out extremely intense movement experiences that often compromised the safety of her body, such as swinging too high and climbing to the top of a tree without any means of getting down. Her thresholds for this input seemed insatiable, and her sensation seeking was disorganized. Her seeking of movement and somatosensory input would often result in an out-of-control high arousal state, exacerbating her emotional outbursts and control-seeking actions. Lola's occupational therapist worked with her in a large sensory gym for 1 hour, three times a week, which allowed her thresholds for movement and somatosensation to be met in a safe, organized manner. Over the course of 3 months, Lola began associating her therapist with these sensory experiences, which felt good for her body, and she slowly began requesting for her therapist to physically help her down from play structures or carry her toward the door in a stretchy blanket when the session ended. Lola continually pushed against boundaries, but her therapist noticed that Lola was more regulated after these boundaries were kindly but firmly consistent: another experience she lacked in her youngest years. Lola was experiencing the sensation of being held by a safe, predictable adult for the first time, which was the first foundational step toward feeling safe in her body and trusting others.

Lola's emerging sense of internal and relational safety fostered an increase of her play level from simple sensorimotor play (climbing, swinging) to constructional, relational play. Lola spontaneously began bringing her therapist into her world by inviting her to sit inside a house she built of blocks, although she continued to need significant control over the play scenario (e.g., dictating what the therapist was to do and say, which blocks to use). Every session, for 10 sessions, Lola's therapist followed her lead in repeatedly building a house, trusting Lola's inner process. One day, Lola requested a new game, suggesting to her therapist that she had resolved a part of her internal struggle to find security. Through play-based sensory experiences with the consistent, steady presence of her therapist,

Lola restructured her narrative from unsafety and unpredictability to an emergent feeling of home. Critically, once Lola began to feel safe with her therapist in the sensory gym, Lola's therapist began to incorporate her foster parent into sessions to work on their relationship through these safe and relational sensorimotor experiences.

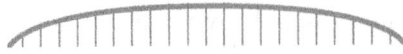

BRIDGING TO PRACTICE 4

When and How Relaxation Exercises May Foster Emotional Shutdown and Feelings of Chronic Helplessness: A Word of Caution

We frequently encounter traumatized individuals who appear numb and emotionally shutdown. Such shutdown states have been associated with an imbalanced ANS, where parasympathetic overdrive is common. Individuals who present chronically shutdown tend to feel persistently depressed, helpless, and emotionally numb. These symptoms are often misunderstood as treatment-resistant depression if not conceptualized from a trauma perspective. Critically, these individuals commonly exhibit blunted activation or arousal to positive or negative stimuli in their lives and hence lose the capacity to feel fully alive. Here, they may feel numb or nothing when their baby smiles at them and reaches out toward them, or, alternatively, they may shut down and be unable to move or fight back when a stranger violates their personal boundaries.

As therapists, we are taught to help our clients engage in relaxation training to calm their chaotic ANS. This can be profoundly helpful when someone exhibits too much arousal and intense emotional states. In this case, relaxation training can soothe sympathetic activation as a means to enhance balance between the sympathetic and parasympathetic branches of the ANS. By stark contrast, when someone is in a chronically numb and shutdown state where they feel depressed and helpless, parasympathetic overdrive is common. By encouraging these individuals to engage in relaxation exercises that target parasympathetic activation, it may instead lead to parasympathetic overdrive and thus exacerbate feelings of emotional shutdown, numbing, depression, and helplessness. In such individuals, activating the sympathetic nervous system in a titrated manner is therefore critical. This can be achieved through activities that raise sympathetic activation and heart rate with the goal of keeping the individual within the window of tolerance. It is crucial that such endeavors involve an *increase* in activity, the antithesis of shutting down, in a personalized manner depending on what an individual can tolerate. Increasing activities that raise sympathetic activation can be akin to activating active defensive responses, which can be safely engaged by walking, pushing against a wall, throwing a ball, kickboxing, or engaging in something that excites a person.

Questions to ask your client:

1. Do you often feel depressed and helpless?
2. Do you feel shutdown?
3. Do you sometimes feel nothing when exposed to pleasurable situations?
4. Do you feel emotionally numb?
5. Does it feel like you are not fully alive?
6. What bodily sensations do you associate with feeling nothing, numb, or not fully alive?
7. Do these feelings make it difficult for you to engage in physical activity?
8. Do these feelings make it difficult for you to engage with others?
9. What happens when you do relaxation exercises? Are you able to connect with your body during relaxation exercises?
10. What happens to your mind and body when you become more physically active?
11. Is there anything your body does automatically to help you overcome feelings of emotional shutdown and helplessness?

Note: You can use your clients' answers to inform the sensory inventory collected from Chapter 1.

Examples of activities that help to activate the sympathetic nervous system:

1. Walking
2. Any form of aerobic exercise (e.g., cycling, running, climbing)
3. Using extensor muscles (e.g., pushing against a wall, reaching for high cabinets, holding antigravity positions)
4. Taking a cold shower
5. Holding an ice cube on the back of the neck
6. Dancing to music
7. Engaging in drumming
8. Doing something that excites an individual

5

Understanding
the Vestibular System

BALANCE, CENTER OF GRAVITY,
AND SEEKING SAFETY AFTER TRAUMA

Movement is the song of the body.
—VANDA SCARAVELLI (1991)

The vestibular system is the most ancient sensory system, dating back through 500 million years of evolution (Graf & Klam, 2006; Smith, 1997). From goldfish to gorillas, all organisms with the capacity to purposefully navigate their environment require a built-in coordinate system. To know our body's position in space requires stimulation from a gravitational pull, orienting us to what is up and what is down, and if and how we are moving. Vestibular input plays a major role in integrating and modulating information from other senses. It's also paramount for effective action, or inaction, in space: For this reason, the vestibular system is the system that never sleeps. The vestibular system is the first system to develop in the womb and, despite being the size of a nickel, acts as an anchor for all other sensory systems in the body.

The vestibular system also orients us during traumatic experiences and may need to be involved in reorienting the brain and body during the healing process. It also engages areas of the brain related to arousal and awareness of inner visceral sensations that guide emotions.

Size Does Not Matter:
How the Smallest Sensory System Carries the Biggest Load

The vestibular organs are located within the inner ear, behind the tympanic membrane dividing the outer and the inner ear. There are two types of sensory receptors located in the vestibular organs: the semicircular canals (anterior, lateral, and posterior) and the otoliths (utricle and saccule), which both respond to the acceleration or deceleration of head movements (Day & Fitzpatrick, 2005; Uchino & Kushiro, 2011). The semicircular canals detect "angular" or rotational movements around the axis of the head, such as nodding (superior canal), tilting toward the shoulder (posterior canal), and shaking your head no (lateral). The head can move in various directions, including up and down, back and forth, and side to side in relation to the downward pull of gravity (see Plate 5.1).

Vestibular information processing varies depending on if head motion is rotary (semicircular canals; i.e., spinning) or linear (otoliths; i.e., back-and-forth movement). The receptors suspended in a gel-like fluid called endolymph can be broken down further into two different-sized hair cells that work in tandem with each other, known as kinocilia and stereocilia. Here, the kinocilia are a stabilizing force that allows the body to maintain its secure base while the stereocilia easily detect and respond to all types of head motion. On top of the gel-like fluid, there are calcium carbonate stones called otoconia (Kingma & van de Berg, 2016). The fluid and otoconia move in response to head motion, creating a deformation in the hair cells that increases or decreases sensory signals to the central vestibular nuclei and cerebellum in the survival brain depending on the direction of head movement. As an example, awakening to a loud crash in the middle of the night requires a posture change involving neck extension to lift the head off the pillow and scan the environment, thereby increasing vestibular signals sent to the otoliths in the inner ear. In contrast, a withdrawn, flexed, and collapsed posture in response to a shaming comment from a parental figure relaxes the neck and back extensors and decreases vestibular signals to the otoliths, perhaps leaving you without a reference point to a secure base and disrupting your center of gravity.

These pathways are linked to autonomic arousal, where hypotonia (or low muscle engagement and tone) is linked with decreased arousal, and hypertonia (characterized by extension against gravity and high muscle engagement and tone) is linked with increased arousal. Vestibular information is intricately connected to the reticular activating system of the survival brain to quickly and preconsciously register any perturbation to postural control and balance, such that disruptions will sharply increase arousal until the body finds solid ground. For example, if one trips over the sidewalk while running, their heart rate increases, pupils dilate, and the appropriate extensor muscles engage until physical equilibrium is restored. This illustrates the intimate connection between arousal and the vestibular system.

Since balance and bodily control are critical to feeling safe in the world, humans are constantly swaying to maintain balance, most often at a subconscious level, which occurs when sitting, standing, walking, or even sleeping. This postural swaying is like your heartbeat in that it is a constant presence but varies in speed and rigor. In terms of the vestibular system, the otoliths are constantly detecting these natural movements to maintain balance and help anchor humans to the earth, thus being a critical factor for embodiment (see Figure 5.1). The connection between the self and the earth is one of the most fundamental relationships in human existence, forming the basis of our essence while still in the womb. The fetus is first passively moved by mother, engendering the first sense of interpersonal connection with vestibular stimulation as the conduit. Ultimately, the integration of vestibular information into our multisensory experience grounds us on our terrain, without which we would be constantly worried about our bodily safety and unable to attend to anything outside of ourselves. In relationships, vestibular stimulation is ever present as we fortify deep bonds with others, from being rocked by a primary caregiver to salsa dancing with a lover. Importantly, the primary attachment relationship and center of gravity are inextricably linked in that they are both dependent upon a secure base to freely explore the surroundings and are vital to shaping one's perception of the inner and outer world.

While the vestibular system translates sensory information to vestibular nuclei in the survival brain via the vestibulocochlear cranial nerve VIII, vestibular information is also intimately connected with the cerebellum, which receives vestibular information both directly and indirectly via the vestibular nuclei. The cerebellum

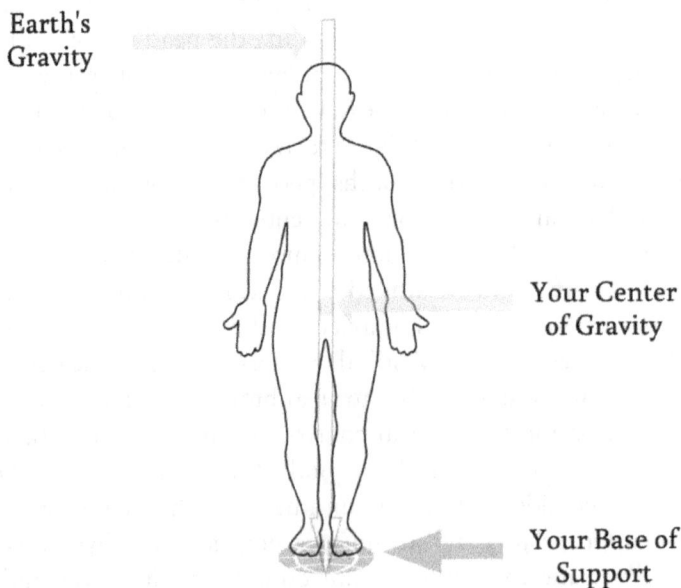

Earth's Gravity

Your Center of Gravity

Your Base of Support

FIGURE 5.1. From stability to agency: anchoring your body in space.

is well-known for its role in motor control and for strengthening one's center of gravity, where body weight is balanced between the upper and lower body. Vestibular information contributes to an overall internal model of gravity, which is said to be created through the interaction and integration of vestibular, proprioceptive, visual, and interoceptive systems (Gallagher, Kearney, & Ferrè, 2021; Harris, 2011; Lacquaniti et al., 2014; Trousselard, Barraud, Nougier, Raphel, & Cian, 2004). Together, the vestibular nuclei and cerebellum engage in a process called *vestibular coding*, where responses to sensory stimuli are used as models when responding to future similar situational demands.

Development, Grounding, and Strategies for Movement

Vestibular coding is initiated when a baby is born, where external and internal sensory input at the level of the survival brain generate automatic, reflexive motor responses as they are not immediately able to control their movements. For example, if a mother's nipple, pacifier, or bottle is used as tactile stimulation on the baby's cheek, the baby will reflexively engage their neck muscles to orient their head toward this and may instinctually reach for it as a source of sustenance and comfort. As more sensory opportunities arise, these reflexive movements start to become consciously initiated as the reflective brain develops and the baby starts to detect the fundamental connection between gravity and successfully navigating the world. In fact, by 5 months, babies start to notice the earth's gravitational pull by expecting that an object thrown in the air will come down, before they can walk or speak. From a sensory point of view, this may explain why a baby seeing a bubble pop when blown into the air evokes a sense of curiosity and surprise, as it defies the baby's expectation for it to fall to the ground. Through these simple experiences and many prediction errors, the baby eventually develops into a toddler who benefits from their newfound stability and begins to experience a sense of agency, feeling secure enough in their postural control and balance to reach for a toy and play with it (and loudly demand that toy you took away).

A child's center of gravity solidifies as they grow older; they feel securely grounded to the earth yet in mastery of their body against its gravitational pull. Interestingly, limited opportunities for free play in children have recently been associated with heightened anxious states in children (Gray, Lancy, & Bjorklund, 2023). This can occur when parents are very risk averse, as they restrict their children from any free play that piques their own curiosity, thus taking away the child's capacity for independence and agency. Consequently, children would be prevented from experiencing prediction errors that are vital to learning about how to navigate balance and establish a strong sense of agency. Unfortunately, the removal of playgrounds in schools for fear of children getting injured comes at the expense of their freedom to play, their trust in their bodies, and their subsequent feeling of safety in the world.

While the vestibular system is essential for establishing one's center of gravity, it also provides a platform for other sensory systems to collaborate with one another to navigate the world. For example, when one's capacity for maintaining their center of gravity is threatened while standing, the central nervous system instinctively acquires information from the vestibular, visual, tactile (from under the feet), and proprioceptive (ankle) information to generate a reactive postural adjustment strategy that helps maintain balance. These strategies are developed over the course of many years of maintaining one's upright posture and center of gravity over many types of terrain (e.g., tiles, grass, sand). Opportunity for movement is crucial for repeated practice using balance-related and postural challenges; these foundational multisensory integrative experiences are prerequisites for future efficacy and efficiency in complex motor actions. Of interest, hip and shoulder muscles, which contribute to a defensive posturing stance, have been anecdotally described by trauma patients as frequently tense. From a biomechanic point of view, this defensive posturing and reactive postural adjustment strategy utilize the same muscle groups, suggesting a link between defensive posturing and the vestibular system.

The Silent Operator: The Subconscious Vestibular System

The vestibular system operates subconsciously, meaning that it is responsible for consistently monitoring our body position and balance without our need to be aware of it. It acts as a silent operator to maintain physical balance and optimal muscle tone as it relies on continuous incoming gravitational information, integrated with sensory input from both the inner body and outside world, to inform body position. This contributes to the body's ability to maintain its center of gravity over a base of support. While the vestibular system has traditionally been viewed to be most heavily implicated in balance, it also plays a determinant role in processing proprioceptive information, including the perception or awareness of the position and movement of the body's muscles and joints.

Most vestibular functions are imperceptible but are still integral for all aspects of engagement with the world, such as balance, posture, stabilizing gaze, spatial awareness, mental rotation for perspective taking, and navigating the environment. Moreover, vestibular sensations can be combined with signals from other sensory systems to aid with their processing.

For example, imagine that you're walking through the woods when you encounter a snake. You need to cross a small stream using a narrow wooden plank to evade it. Vestibular input provides the information necessary to maintain your center of gravity and balance while walking across the plank. It also contributes toward the heightening of your muscle tone in reference to gravitational pull to allow a more rigid and controlled stance in response to the potential danger of the situation. Your fear of snakes also manifests as a pit in the stomach while you frantically scan your environment for the snake. In order to cross the plank and get to safety successfully, the vestibular system utilizes additional visual, proprioceptive, and interoceptive sensations to see the plank; avoid the snake; and urgently yet precisely navigate across. Importantly, as seen from this example, the vestibular system orchestrates the other senses in reference to the body's actions as it modulates and coordinates other sensory systems to help navigate one's internal and external worlds. It can be viewed as a stabilizing force that allows all sensory systems to work in synchrony.

Notably, vestibular dysfunction in humans is often associated with anxiety disorders, including panic attacks and phobias, as well as depression. Serotonin receptors are found in the vestibular nerve and vestibular nucleus, but the functional significance of this remains uncertain (Ahn & Balaban, 2010). While it is possible that anxiety is a direct consequence of vestibular dysfunction, it has also been reported that anxiety disorders can cause dizziness of vestibular origin (Asmundson, Norton, Allerdings, Norton, & Larsen, 1998; Best et al., 2006; Bolmont, Gangloff, Vouriot, & Perrin, 2002; Furman & Marcus, 2012; Staab, Ruckenstein, Solomon, & Shepard, 2002; Tecer, Tukel, Erdamar, & Sunay, 2004; Venault et al., 2001). In addition, antidepressants, such as selective serotonin reuptake inhibitors, have been reported to relieve dizziness associated with psychiatric disorders. However, Halberstadt and Balaban (2006) showed that the dorsal raphe nucleus in the survival brain releases serotonin and communicates with the vestibular nuclei in the survival brain and the amygdala in the emotional learning brain. This finding suggests that vestibular dysfunction may be related to a multitude of changes in emotion processing and that changes in emotion and physical balance may be intimately linked, paving an important path of inquiry into vestibular processing alterations in the aftermath of trauma.

Binding Our External and Internal Worlds: How Vestibular Sensory Information Travels through the Brain

Vestibular sensory information derived from the semicircular canals and otoliths in the inner ear first travels to the vestibular nuclei in the brainstem and the fastigial nucleus of the most ancient aspect of the cerebellum, the bulb within the base of the brain that is integral for a host of functions such as coordinating movement. The vestibular nuclei and the fastigial nucleus are the foundational base of primary vestibular processing; it is here that vestibular information first integrates with proprioceptive input to inform the individual of the position of the head and neck and of the origin of motion ("Am I moving or am I being moved?"). Information from the vestibular nuclei and cerebellum is then directed for additional processing to the emotional learning and reflective brain sections. Information about the position of the head and neck in space are sent to higher-order regions of the brain for more advanced processing to guide movement and foster a conscious understanding of where the head and body are in the context of one's environment. Herein is another example of how the base of the brain, which receives incoming sensory information, is vital for directing how information is processed at higher levels of the brain and is therefore a lynchpin for the reintegration of the self after trauma.

Simultaneously, vestibular information also integrates with interoceptive sensory information through the reticular activating system, a hub in the survival brain critical for the modulation of arousal. Here, the reticular activating system is a common entry point for interoceptive pathways from the body, including pain, temperature, and visceral sensations from the vagus nerve (discussed in Chapter 6). The reticular activating system interacts intimately with the periaqueductal gray to coordinate the fight-or-flight response, freezing/tonic immobility, and the emotional shutdown/withdrawal response (see Chapter 4). It is at this lower half of the survival brain where raw affect, arousal, and sensation meet, which is where and how the insult of trauma is first detected in the brain and then mapped onto the vestibular system.

The vestibular nuclei in the survival brain then make connections with the thalamus in the emotional learning brain (Cullen & Chacron, 2023). As we saw in Chapter 4, the thalamus acts as a vital gateway for transmitting sensory information to the cortex. It can be a line of demarcation in the brain between the subcortex (emotional learning and survival brain sections) and the cortex (the reflective brain). Specifically, *vestibular thalamocortical neurons*, those that transmit vestibular information through the thalamus to the cortex, differentiate passive motion from voluntary movements, thus mediating our sense of agency or ability to act on the environment (Cullen & Chacron, 2023; Lopez & Blanke, 2011). Overall, the thalamus acts as an access point for connection to higher sections of the brain, allowing an individual to gain a deeper understanding of where their body is in space. Importantly, vestibular thalamocortical connections not only encode information about bodily orientation and motion but also regarding arousal (reviewed in Lopez & Blanke, 2011). This may help coordinate postural shifts toward a more defensive stance in response to heightened arousal. The vestibular input also uses its connections with the hippocampus to provide a frame of reference for spatial memory, which defines where the person was in the environment when an event occurred. Critically, it is important to think about out-of-body responses during a traumatic event, where the individual has no reference to where they are in time and space, which then disrupts their capacity to encode and later recall spatial memory (Bergouignan et al., 2014, 2022).

The Balance System: Knowing Where, Why, and How to Move

Beyond the thalamus, there are vestibular processing hubs in the reflective brain, including the temporoparietal junction (TPJ), the posterior insula, and the surrounding parietal operculum, which are all involved in integrating sensations from the external and internal worlds. Specifically, these areas have been identified as critical for the underpinning neurobiology of trauma, thus emphasizing the importance of the vestibular system's contributions toward healing the traumatized brain. We discuss each area in depth below.

Knowing Where to Move: The Hub for Processing the External World

The TPJ, a critical hub for processing external sensations, lies where the temporal and parietal lobes meet on each side of the reflective brain. The TPJ works in close association with the parietal operculum, particularly the subregion known as OP2, which has been identified in humans to be a core hub for processing vestibular sensations (Ibitoye et al., 2023; zu Eulenburg, Caspers, Roski, & Eickhoff, 2012). This area is thought to be critical for defining the self both physically and mentally, such as how we understand boundaries of the self in space and how the self is differentiated from others. It is a hub for many of the key networks in the brain, including those involved with understanding where one is in space (i.e., visuospatial processing) and how individuals meaningfully connect with others (e.g., theory of mind). Part of one's ability to connect with others and experience empathy is grounded in the capacity to mentally rotate one's perspective to take that of another. Here, vestibular information is critical for performing geometrical transformations, such as translations and rotations, of one's viewpoint (Deroualle, Borel, Deveze, & Lopez, 2015; Mast, Merfeld, & Kosslyn, 2006; van Elk & Blanke, 2014; for a review, see Deroualle & Lopez, 2014).

In support of these notions, the TPJ has been shown to be involved in out-of-body experiences, where an individual perceives that they are separate from, and sometimes floating above and looking down upon, their physical body (Blanke & Arzy, 2005). This implication of the TPJ in this phenomenon is particularly relevant for trauma-related dissociation given the profound sense of detachment from the body experienced, often to the point of not knowing where one begins or ends. This information is crucial in understanding where one is in space, which is needed to know *where* to move in response to sensory information in an individual's surroundings.

Knowing Why to Move: The Insula as a Hub for Processing the Internal World

The insula, an area tucked just underneath the prefrontal cortex toward the brain's core, is a critical hub for processing both vestibular information and internal sensations from the body (Baier et al., 2013). Given the intimate connections between the vestibular nuclei and the insula, we propose that the vestibular system provides the foundation for interoception. It is nestled beneath the parietal operculum, a key vestibular processing and multisensory integrative region. The insula is a key region for many different neural networks, including those involved with interoception, attention, pain processing, and emotion identification. The insula can be subdivided into two separate areas, including the posterior insula (back of the insula) and the anterior insula (front of the insula).

The posterior insula maintains neural connections to both the brainstem in the survival brain and the amygdala in the emotional learning brain, where it receives sensory information about raw affect, arousal, and visceral sensations from the inner body. The posterior insula is key in processing these interoceptive sensations, including those related to pain, pressure, arousal, hunger, thirst, and temperature. The posterior insula, along with the parietal operculum, is also a key part of what is known as the "vestibular cortex"—a poorly delineated brain area involved in cortical vestibular processing in humans (zu Eulenburg, Stephan, Dieterich, & Ruehl, 2020). (This region is known as the parieto-insular vestibular cortex in primates; see Akbarian et al., 1988.)

The posterior insula transfers integrated vestibular-interoceptive information to the anterior portion of the insula to identify the relevant emotions. For example, if a visceral sensation originating from the stomach is identified as fullness and bloating in the posterior insula, the anterior insula would interpret it as a signal to stop eating and may cue a host of emotions depending on one's context and belief systems (satisfaction, shame). Here, understanding the interoceptive and physiological context from inner visceral sensations allows an individual to understand *why* they should move or act in response to sensory information.

Knowing How to Move: Integrating the External and Internal Worlds in the Reflective Brain

Imagine guiding a frail loved one down a flight of stairs, and they fall to the ground. Think about the emotions that it would evoke. Maybe you are imagining a pit in your stomach, or a sinking feeling. This sensation may be translated to fear or panic, contributing to your understanding of *why* you want (or need) to move. The vestibular system helps you understand where you are, how you are postured in reference to your loved one, and then engages the appropriate extensor musculature to quickly act. This type of sensory input references three-dimensional space, allowing for the mental rotation required to see the situation from their perspective, eliciting visceral feelings of anguish and discomfort. This illustrates how the external and internal worlds work in tandem within the vestibular system to allow an individual to decide how to move: to move with agency and to experience empathetic sensations.

As described above, information relayed to the TPJ, the parietal operculum, and the posterior insula about sensory information related to the external world and the internal body is then translated to cortical networks, which consolidates to form a unified sensory perspective that facilitates curiosity, exploration, and reflection. This process allows the individual to experience the body as a coherent, stable entity that exists in the present. Furthermore, it fosters the feeling that one is connected with and grounded in the world, facilitating an embodied state of strong mind and body connection.

When Fear Tips You Over: The Vestibular System after Trauma

One of the most fundamental human relationships is one's relationship to the gravitational field of the earth (Ayres & Robbins, 2005). The experience of trauma frequently leaves individuals without a firm center of gravity and instead with an insecure and fallible connection to the earth, thereby gutting their foundational sense of safety in the body (Harricharan et al., 2017, 2021; Kearney & Lanius, 2022). As one traumatized individual noted, "I often feel off balance, so I can't feel safe in the world." The vestibular/balance system is integral in fortifying this foundational sense of gravitational safety, a basic human need that often cannot be fully met in the aftermath of trauma.

Attachment disruptions are often the origin of a mal-developed grounding to the earth, where stimulation of the vestibular/balance system did not occur with a safe caregiver. The result is a paucity or absence of opportunities to be rocked, cuddled, and swirled about due to their caregivers' own struggles. Furthermore, traumatized children often grow up in terror, where the sole means of survival is to focus on threat, thus depriving them of the ability to freely play and explore the world. Exploration and play are critical activities for optimal development of this balance system and help strengthen one's center of gravity for a firm and safe grounding to this planet.

Anecdotally, traumatized individuals are frequently left feeling as though they are "floating" without a firm connection to the ground, thus leaving them vulnerable and open to attack. Indeed, a traumatized individual noted, "I had no center of gravity, no ballast. I had no center at all. I was easily influenced by the company I was in or the movie I'd just seen, easily shaken, knocked off my feet." These feelings of imbalance can be exacerbated further when the individual is reminded of their trauma. As mentioned above, a traumatized individual stated, "When I'm triggered, there is just a small emotion that explodes throughout my whole body and causes me to freeze. When I freeze, I feel the imbalance and start tilting to one side." These first-person experiences outline elegantly the critical implications of vestibular processing in the aftermath of trauma.

In this section, we discuss the emerging clinical and neurobiological evidence that illustrates how the vestibular (balance) system is profoundly affected by trauma, which can leave the individual feeling uprooted, ungrounded, and unable to move safely through their environment (Harricharan et al., 2017, 2021; Kearney & Lanius, 2022). This, in turn, can have a significant impact on how the traumatized individual perceives their inner and external worlds.

Studies of individuals who were not suffering from PTSD or any other emotional difficulties provide a good comparison. As several groups have reported (Pfeiffer, Serino, & Blanke, 2014), the vestibular nuclei in the survival brain, which receives information from the balance system in the inner ear, has important connections with brain regions that are critical to the perception of the inner body and the external environment, specifically the posterior insula, parietal operculum, and the TPJ (as described above). These regions also maintain connections with the prefrontal cortex, where information from the internal and external worlds is integrated to inform abstract thinking, agency to engage with the world, sense of the present, social connection, and the feeling of being alive through embodiment. Importantly, integration of the information of the internal and external worlds at the level of the prefrontal cortex also integrates this information with past experiences, which allows an individual to reflect on how one's current experience may relate to the past and formulate a coherent narrative to interpret the current experience. Last, a recent study using high-field-strength magnetic resonance imaging (MRI) found that the vestibular nuclei have strong connections with the brain's default mode network (DMN), further bolstering the notion that vestibular processing contributes to one's sense of self and their relationship to the past, present, and future (Cauzzo et al., 2022; see also Rabellino et al., 2023).

Among individuals affected by trauma, the brain structures involved in the vestibular (balance) system are uniquely affected. A recent study from our group examined these effects in two groups of individuals who suffer from PTSD, including those who experience severe out-of-body experiences as seen in the dissociative subtype of PTSD, and those who experience dissociation to a lesser degree and more predominantly exhibit hyperarousal and hypervigilance symptoms (known as the PTSD group; Harricharan et al., 2017). The findings were strikingly different between the two groups.

Individuals in the PTSD group, who experience less marked dissociative symptoms, demonstrated weakened connections between the vestibular nucleus in the survival brain and the posterior insula, the brain region involved in registering one's internal state of the body. This may suggest that individuals with PTSD have more difficulties registering vestibular signals and integrating these with input from the internal world of their body, perhaps leading to intense, unbearable visceral feeling states (reviewed in Harricharan et al., 2021; Kearney & Lanius, 2022). In the PTSD group, the vestibular nuclei also showed increased connection to the TPJ, the part of the brain critical for defining the boundary between self and other, which is a vital process for engendering a sense of body ownership. This increased connection among individuals with PTSD suggests that these individuals are hyperfocused on the external environment and their orientation within it, thus preparing for threat and perpetuating a sustained experience of hypervigilance and hyperarousal symptoms. This may explain why vestibular stimulation by sitting in a rocking chair or a sensory hammock among individuals with PTSD may reduce hypervigilance symptoms, as they utilize calming vestibular stimulation to decrease arousal and increase connection to the earth that may, in turn, shift connectivity patterns in the brain. This phenomenon can often be observed among traumatized individuals who rock back and forth in a rhythmic pattern to soothe themselves.

Individuals who suffer from PTSD and exhibit prominent out-of-body responses showed starkly contrasting patterns of brain connections involving the vestibular nuclei of the survival brain. These individuals showed significantly decreased connections between the vestibular nuclei and the TPJ, suggesting a diminished ability to register the external world, maintain body ownership, or know where the body is in space. In addition, limited connections were observed between the vestibular nuclei and the prefrontal cortex in the reflective brain, suggesting that information about the inner body and the external environment are not optimally integrated. This makes it difficult to form a unified sensory experience or remain aware of the body's movements and positioning. For example, intense bodily sensations crop up without appropriate context of their origin, manifesting as unbearable visceral feeling states that are perceived as an inescapable threat that makes the individual feel helpless. In other words, if one feels disconnected from one's own body, it makes it difficult to interact with their surroundings and establish ownership and agency over their actions, thus perpetuating the sense of being estranged and disconnected from the world.

CASE EXAMPLE: Suzy—"When I Close My Eyes, I Don't Know Where I Am"

Suzy is a 55-year-old woman who suffered severe childhood trauma. All that she knew, and thus her only source of comfort, was her relationship with her perpetrator. Even though Suzy is incredibly resilient and creative, which has aided her healing, she continues to struggle to maintain a strong center of gravity that keeps her grounded. Interestingly, her therapist noted that she frequently reports "I don't know where I am when I close my eyes." Suzy's medical history was known to her therapist, and she confirmed that she had no muscular or neurological diseases. Given her clinical presentation, it can be speculated that Suzy cannot process vestibular information in a manner that adequately registers and integrates sensory cues from the external world, thereby preventing her from understanding where her body is in space. Here, we postulate that she compensates for disrupted vestibular processing by relying primarily on visual input to feel anchored and connected to her surroundings. However, this comes at the great cost of never truly feeling centered in her own vessel. To test these clinical observations, a medical professional performed several standardized neurological tests of vestibular function on Suzy, none of which required equipment.

The Romberg Test

This test involves having the person stand up with their feet together for up to 30 seconds with their eyes open and then closed while varying their own center of gravity (e.g., feet placed heel-to-toe) or center of gravity (e.g., arms crossed over chest while holding their shoulders). If a clear sway is observed or the person loses their stance, this indicates a Romberg sign, suggestive of impairment in either vestibular, cerebellar, or proprioceptive function.

When standing with eyes open, Suzy was able to maintain all positions for the duration of 30 seconds. However, when doing the test with her eyes closed, standing with her feet side by side, she showed increased sway, with a loss of balance and her head shifting from its initial position. More importantly, Suzy's eyes tightened shut, and her face contorted in a terrified manner. Given her dysregulation in the previous test, she was not able to perform the test in the heel-to-toe stance. However, it was evident that Suzy's vestibular system was not operating adequately without the use of visual input to anchor her in space.

The Smooth Tracking Test

The extraocular eye muscles help the eyes orient our bodies to the environment. Despite their small size, these extraocular eye muscles are utilized more than the arm and chest muscles for balance because we are constantly engaging them in response to our surroundings. Because the vestibular nuclei are imperative for eliciting eye movements, smooth tracking is frequently used to test the extraocular muscles' function and integration with the vestibular system. Smooth tracking involves the clinician holding a finger about 12 inches (30 cm) from the participant's face while engaging them in smooth pursuit eye movements horizontally, vertically, and diagonally, followed by bringing the finger close to the face to see the eyes converge.

When this test was administered to Suzy, she was not able to fully follow the smooth pursuit eye movement horizontally and vertically, where her eyes came back quickly to the center and could not extend to both sides. Also, she showed synkinesis (e.g., unintentional muscle contraction in the face) while moving her eyes, where her mouth moved in tandem with her eye movements even though it was not solicited. When testing eye convergence, Suzy was unable to bring her eyes together and showed lip twitching. Finally, Suzy mentioned feeling fatigued due to muscle strain in her eyes from the test.

Finger-to-Nose Test

Upper-limb coordination involves use of the cerebellum, which, among its many roles, serves as a hub of interaction between proprioceptive, visual, vestibular, and tactile input. A classic neurological test is the "finger-to-nose test," where the client extends one arm out in front of them while isolating the index finger and uses their other hand to repeatedly touch the extended index finger and then their nose back and forth. Repetition should yield improvement, and fluidity should be observed due to enhanced motor coordination over time spent doing the test.

When this test was administered to Suzy, her movements were jerky and she was unable to touch her finger while doing the test with her eyes closed.

Suzy's case illustrates recent evidence that symptoms seen in classic neurological disorders following stroke or head trauma may also occur in the aftermath of emotional trauma. Her therapist incorporated strategies to engage her vestibular system at her own pace, and Suzy was able to improve her emotional and physical equilibrium.

How Movement during Therapy Restores the Center of Gravity

The traditional therapeutic setting involves sitting in a chair in an office, facing the therapist. The individual is tasked with discussing trauma-related beliefs and associated strategies to challenge them and/or engage in exposure to feared events. Although many adults can participate in therapy through these methods, it may not be tolerable for some. Furthermore, children have a difficult time regulating themselves enough to sit still throughout a therapy session. Critically, however, both populations experience disruptions to sensory processing, including vestibular processing. Given that both adults and children frequently suffer from feeling off balance and insecure in their bodies, how should we think about addressing these difficulties in the therapeutic environment?

A key therapeutic strategy that stimulates the vestibular system is rhythmic motion, which involves moving back and forth at a steady pace to create a stable internal reference point that the body can use to anchor itself in space. Rhythm essentially facilitates synchrony between the mind and body, where repetitive, predictable movements can elicit a soothing effect and calm arousal. Rhythm stimulates the vestibular nuclei, reticular formation, and the cerebellum, which have calming, regulating impacts on the upper sections of the brain.

Although adults can tolerate the traditional therapeutic environment, it may not allow for the optimal brain–body dialogue vital for dynamic engagement with one's self and others. Instead of a traditional therapeutic environment, the client may be better served if the therapist creates a safe space that encourages movement and physical balance through different postures to activate the vestibular system, including but not limited to an aerial yoga swing, a rocking chair, an exercise ball, or a balance board (Champagne, 2011; Mullen et al., 2008). The application of these strategies in trauma treatment for children and adolescents has been championed by Elizabeth Warner and her team in Boston, Massachusetts, where they have developed a therapeutic intervention called sensory motor arousal regulation therapy (SMART; Warner et al., 2020). SMART is a neuroscientifically guided treatment that allows traumatized individuals to discover their personalized sensory needs and thresholds, which, in turn, facilitates restoration of physical balance, regulation of emotions, formation of trauma narratives, exploration of their internal and external worlds, and connection with their loved ones.

The SMART therapeutic paradigm relies on sensory–motor engagement through the combined effect of the therapeutic relationship and basic sensory equipment that challenge and optimize the most fundamental relationship between oneself and the earth. By fostering a tangible anchor to the ground, vestibular input within SMART sessions can promote a safer and more stable bond between child and caregiver, opening the gateway for connection and belonging. This approach has the potential to be utilized beyond the therapeutic setting and can be incorporated into community programming, schools, foster and group homes, detention centers, and correctional facilities. This intervention is unique in that it emphasizes the cultivation of stability in both the mental and physical realms as opposed to focusing solely on the cognitive and affect-related processes placed at the center of traditional therapeutic approaches. By engaging both the mental and physical aspects of the individual, it maximizes one's capacity to overcome the profound brain, mind, and body disconnect that is at the core of trauma-related suffering (Bridging to Practice 5 offers some additional guidance to implement these strategies in a therapeutic setting).

CASE EXAMPLE: Jarred—Coming Alive with Vestibular Stimulation

Jarred was 14 years old when his parents brought him to therapy. His symptoms included excessive hand washing to the point of scarring, and he reported hearing sounds when no sound was present. He was placed under suicide watch at the hospital for 48 hours after his parents found a rope in his room and he subsequently revealed a plan to kill himself. During his hospitalization, Jarred was diagnosed with psychosis not yet defined. Afterward, Jarred disclosed to his parents that he had been repeatedly bullied at school for the past 2 years, including having his lunch money stolen and being the target of a barrage of offensive slurs (e.g., "maggot," "girlie boy," "cockroach"). When his parents spoke to the therapist, they mentioned that Jarred had shifted from a curious teen to being highly anxious and distressed approximately 1 month prior to his hospitalization. Following his hospitalization, Jarred had spent a week in his bed, still not his former self. His parents brought him for outpatient therapy 10 days later.

During his first session, Jarred exhibited a slouched posture, limited eye contact, and grayish skin (this clinical presentation is consistent with the dissociative emotional shutdown response discussed in the defense cascade model from Chapter 4). His speech was monotone, and he endorsed feeling as though he was "floating in space" and "felt the ground was not under me." He also reported that he wished he had taken his own life, as he could not find pleasure in being in proximity of other people, including his own family. During parent consultation, Jarred's parents mentioned that he used to enjoy swinging in the park growing up. The therapist decided to use a SMART approach, which included setting up a hammock swing in the therapy room.

Vestibular Activation as an Anchor

When Jarred entered the room, he naturally gravitated toward the swing. Jarred did not initiate swinging until his therapist asked if it would be okay if they gently moved the swing. Only then did he initiate movement, which seemed enough to foster curiosity toward the sensation. He started off gently tilting in the swing and gradually progressed to fully swinging over the span of 45 minutes. Notably, the therapist inquired about where Jarred would like them to be in the room and Jarred asked them to stand in the corner. With more robust swinging, he started to giggle, and his posture became more erect, although he was still not able to make eye contact with the therapist. In subsequent sessions, the therapist followed Jarred's pace as he continued to seek gentle vestibular stimulation to anchor himself (e.g., rocking back and forth on the swing) at a steady rhythm. He eventually started opening up to the therapist and explained that his bullies threatened that they would kill him if he told anyone about the bullying. He also mentioned that he had been repeatedly bullied throughout his life and coped by creating a "better world in my mind" that he would escape to [in his emotional shutdown state]. While swinging and telling his story, Jarred was able to engage in the type of free movement that had always been lost when he was frozen by the words of his perpetrators. As Jarred activated sensory stimulation at a threshold he was comfortable with—which was gently suggested by his therapist (swinging Jarred in different planes and monitoring his reactions)—Jarred was able to verbalize his felt sensations in his stomach and his heart space.

Orienting to the Caregiver: Vestibular Stimulation
Leads to Insular Activation and Access to Language and Emotions

Although Jarred tried out different sensory equipment, he always defaulted to swinging. At baseline his body felt numb, but he noticed that he felt an urge to connect with his parents after he swung. His numbness had been preventing him from feeling emotionally connected and soothed by his mother. Jarred was only able to feel an inkling of connection with his mother during intense arguments. His therapist suggested they invite his mother into the therapy room. Before going into the session, the therapist suggested to Jarred's mother that she allow Jarred to initiate contact and to not force him to talk unless he wanted to. The therapist suspected that Jarred would open up emotionally on his own if the mother modeled an open, nonjudgmental stance. The mother entered the room and sat diagonally to the swing that Jarred sat in. Jarred started to swing and immediately oriented to face his mother.[1] They engaged in the following dialogue:

JARRED (J): I remember I really liked to swing when I was young. I wonder why I ever stopped. Oh yeah (*sulks*), I remember now, it was because of these boys. They made me think I don't deserve to feel any pleasure.

MOTHER (M): (*softly*) Oh Jarred, I'm so sorry I was not able to be there for you. I just wish you could know that all I ever want is for my children to be happy. How hard that must have been for you to think this.

J: I know, mama, I just did not want to bother you with my things. You had so much on your plate with the adoption of my sister.

M: Jarred, I am always there for you anytime you need me. You matter so much and all that I want is to do anything so that you are happy.

Jarred then gently brought his swinging to a halt and extended his head to fully look at his mother. His eyes started to water.

J: (*Sighs.*) I hate these boys, and I wished it never happened.

M: I do too, baby.

Jarred's mom approached him and they hugged. After a good cry, Jarred went back to swinging but wanted his mother to push the swing. Before this interaction, neither Jarred nor his mother or therapist had realized the deep instability he had experienced when his parents adopted his sister, which likely contributed to his sense of disconnection to his primary regulatory anchors in his earlier years.

After 10 sessions, Jarred began setting up activities to complete during his session, such as balance obstacles and self-guided swinging. The active, agentive engagement in purposeful movement fostered communication with himself and his own body, which eventually culminated in him feeling connected enough to retell his story to his parents. Outside of sessions, he gradually started to engage in social outings that incorporated movement as per his therapist's suggestion, including bowling events with a local nursing home. Despite wanting to push himself to speed up his progress, the therapist emphasized the importance of treatment proceeding at a tolerable pace that feels safe to him. Fortunately, Jarred viewed his home as a safe place and created a space in his bedroom with a cushion on the floor (to initiate slight instability requiring balance) and an exercise ball to move in different directions. This space served as his anchor to stay grounded.

---

[1] It is crucial to note that, as the vestibular system is activated through different directions, an ideal therapy space should have a swing that permits easy 360-degree movement around a swivel as spontaneous actions may occur.

During his later sessions, Jarred started to regularly stand with an upright posture, better articulate his needs, and set boundaries with his parents and his peers. Interestingly, the therapist spotted Jarred in public several years later and saw him smiling during a walk with his spouse, clearly basking in the fresh air of fall.

The slower you go, the faster you get there.
—RICHARD KLUFT (1993)

Notably, an intervention that incorporates rhythmicity is eye movement desensitization and reprocessing (EMDR), which involves recalling traumatic memories while simultaneously engaging in rhythmic eye movements or alternating bilateral stimulation to reduce vividness and emotional potency of traumatic memories (Shapiro, 1989; Shapiro & Maxfield, 2002). The simultaneous bilateral stimulation allows for in-depth visuospatial reconstruction of the memory, which intersects with key reflective brain areas involved in integrating vestibular input with exteroceptive sensations, such as the TPJ (Kavanagh, Freese, Andrade, & May, 2001; Landin-Romero, Moreno-Alcazar, Pagani, & Amann, 2018; Maxfield, Melnyk, & Hayman, 2008; Pagani, Högberg, Fernandez, & Siracusano, 2013). In addition, Harricharan and colleagues (2019) showed that bilateral eye movements activate the anterior insula, a key structure for interoception and vestibular–somatosensory integration. Theoretical postulations about EMDR propose that bilateral sensory stimulation during traumatic memory recall synchronizes networks critical to the perception of our inner and outer worlds, shaping the emotional tone of the memory at the level of the dorsolateral prefrontal cortex in the reflective brain (Lanius, Paulsen, & Corrigan, 2014; Rousseau et al., 2019) and, potentially, eye movement and/or somatosensory processing centers in the survival brain. Vestibular stimulation through rhythmic eye movements is also thought to contribute to the integration of sensorimotor, autobiographical memory, social connection, and emotion regulation neural networks in the brain and alleviate the effects of trauma (Bergmann, 2008; Harricharan et al., 2019).

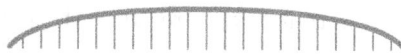

BRIDGING TO PRACTICE 5

The Silent Choreographer:
The Vestibular System as an Orchestrator of Equilibrium

As vestibular input informs us that our head and body are in motion, it directs our attention to the physical body to ensure we maintain our orientation, balance, and equilibrium, anchoring us in time and space. It is also a powerful modulator of arousal. Oftentimes, we incorporate vestibular input intuitively into our daily lives to enhance body awareness and regulate arousal. Think of a time in the recent past where you felt stressed or anxious. What did you do? Can you think of any movement-based behaviors or activities that you've used to calm your nerves? Some common examples can include pacing while on a stressful phone call, walking or running, bike riding, driving, or rocking back and forth. Alternatively, what is something you do when you're feeling low arousal and need to remain alert? Perhaps you get up and get a cup of coffee. Although the caffeine may be the most obvious stimulant here, the activity of getting up and going for a walk can help us become more alert and organized due to the vestibular (and proprioceptive) feedback we receive. Some may need higher levels of stimulation to feel within an optimal arousal zone, such as intense physical exercise or fast driving. For therapists, this vestibular awareness exercise can be done with your clients to help in understanding the concept of vestibular input as an arousal regulation and body awareness tool.

Questions to ask your client:

1. What do you do when you're feeling stressed? Does this involve any movements of your head and/or body?
2. What do you do when you're feeling tired and need to remain alert? Does this involve any movements of your head and/or body?
3. How do different planes of movement feel to you? Explore linear (back and forth), rotary (spinning), and orbital (moving in a large circle around a central object).

As a therapeutic tool, vestibular stimulation can be explored and altered to stimulate the different vestibular organs (otoliths vs. semicircular canals) and direct awareness toward the body. For clients with sensory hyperresponsivities to other sensory modalities (touch, auditory), working through the vestibular system (instead of the other sensory systems directly) can have a modulatory effect in reducing these hypersensitivities. To stimulate the different vestibular organs, explore different planes of movement with your client. *Ensure this movement is first self-initiated: The proprioceptive feedback from self-motion is less alerting when first engaging in vestibular exploration.*

Examples of vestibular activities that regulate the nervous system (for hyper- or hypoarousal) include the following:

1. Linear and rhythmic movements, bouncing on a therapy ball, or rocking in a rocking chair
2. Walking
3. Swaying side to side
4. Any form of aerobic exercise with a steady rhythm (e.g., cycling, running)
5. Using extensor muscles (e.g., pushing against a wall, reaching for high cabinets, holding antigravity positions)
6. Dancing to music

7. Engaging in drumming or music (vibrations stimulate the vestibular system)
8. Rotary (spinning) motion, though this is highly individualized

Examples of typically alerting vestibular activities to try with your (hypoaroused) client:

1. Linear acceleration (e.g., on a swing)
2. Nonlinear movements (rotary/spinning or orbital movement)
3. Closing the eyes while on a swing or unstable surface; this has a bigger impact on arousal
4. Imposed movement, such as being moved by another while on a swing or other piece of sensory equipment (ensure the client feels safe within your therapeutic relationship and provides informed consent)
5. Climbing (vestibular–visual detection of being off the ground can be alerting)

6

Interoception and Visceral Sensations after Trauma
THE WAR WITHIN

An organism must be able to experience its own existence
as a sentient being before it can experience the existence
and salience of anything else in the environment.
—ALVIN "BUD" CRAIG (2009)

Interoception can be considered the brain's representation of sensations from within the body, allowing us to answer the question, "How do I feel?" in any given moment. Bud Craig published a seminal paper describing interoception in 2003, defining it as one's perception and understanding of the physiological state of the body, particularly intuiting inner visceral bodily sensations in response to external stimuli in one's environment. Examples of inner visceral sensations include hunger, thirst, arousal, and tickling, as well as sensing a pit in the stomach related to dread or a warm sensation on the chest indicative of joy. These visceral sensations are the primal underpinnings of emotions and influence one's subjective emotional experience—as such, interoceptive experience is profoundly disrupted in psychiatric conditions associated with dysregulated arousal.

Since the start of this book, we have emphasized how adaptive behavior stems from secure attachment relationships early in life, which are first felt through our senses and generate beliefs about safety, or lack thereof, in the world. Maladaptive behavior, or behavior that creates and perpetuates distress for oneself and/or others, may in turn stem from an insecure attachment foundation. In this chapter, we further discuss how inner sensations paint a picture of how we predict and envision the world in the aftermath of trauma, and how they are harnessed to drive our first and foremost imperative: survival. After trauma, inner sensations become primarily oriented to potential threats, generating a perpetual state of terror, chaos, and unpredictability. When we are constantly putting out fires, we don't have time to orient to other, less urgent experiences of calm, joy, or connectedness. As such, persistent hypervigilance comes at the expense of feeling fully alive in the present moment.

Sensing the Inner World of the Body

The interoceptive system engages all sections of the brain (survival brain, emotional learning brain, reflective brain). Many of the brain regions discussed here are also involved in the vestibular system. The vagus nerve is considered a superhighway between the body's internal organs and the survival brain, carrying vital information about inner bodily sensations (Paciorek & Skora, 2020). The reticular activating system is a web-like cluster of neurons in the survival brain that receives input from our various senses as well as areas in the brainstem involved in arousal and raw emotion, including the locus coeruleus and the periaqueductal gray (Magoun, 1952). The reticular activating system is a critical part of the brain involved in generating alertness, and it carries interoceptive sensory information from the inner body and transfers it to upper layers of the brain, where we become consciously aware of what we feel. In the reflective brain, the insula is considered central to this processing of interoceptive sensations and helps identify the emotional feeling states that underpin them. More specifically, the posterior (back) part of the insula receives information about raw visceral sensations from both the survival and emotional learning layers of the brain, while the anterior (front) part looks to identify the emotional feeling states underpinning these visceral sensations.

Many traumatized individuals feel cut off from their inner sensations, unable to dictate or act appropriately on how they feel. For these individuals, this interoceptive pathway must be harnessed to develop a sense of *interoceptive awareness*, which refers to one's own attunement to the sensations of their inner body, thereby facilitating the capacity to inhabit one's own body and make sense of one's feelings.

When Interoception Becomes Unbearable: Disconnecting from One's Inner World of Sensations and Feelings

Early adverse experiences can significantly interfere with one's capacity for interoceptive awareness. When trapped in a dangerous environment, such as being with a neglectful or a physically or sexually abusive caregiver, individuals are prevented from using their inner sensations and "gut feelings" to guide effective actions and behaviors. For example, if a child is in an abusive relationship with a caregiver and has the impulse to escape, they may quickly learn that escape is not possible. A sense of learned helplessness may ensue, as we saw in Chapter 4 when we discussed emotional shutdown as part of the defense cascade. Individuals with such experiences therefore learn that emotional responses to traumatic events are futile because there is no escape. Hence, they become increasingly disconnected from their inner emotional life as a means to cope with intolerable sensations and feelings that seem out of control. This effect is amplified if the child lacks the presence of any attuned caregiver to help them contain and make meaning of these feelings while buffering the intensity of these sensations. Without a road map for navigating trusting relationships, traumatized individuals are frequently left to cycle between unbearable feelings of terror and feelings of emotional numbing. They enter a state of emotional anesthesia that prevents them from feeling as though they fully exist in the present. In this state, traumatized individuals are often unable to feel love toward their partners or children, thus leaving them not only disconnected from themselves but also from their most cherished relationships. This, in turn, can rob the traumatized person of feeling safe in a nurturing relationship, which perpetuates a sense of brokenness and forsakenness in the world.

It is therefore not surprising that traumatized individuals, including persons with PTSD, often exhibit problems being aware of their own emotional states and have difficulties identifying and labeling these states. Studies have shown that these individuals have lower scores on the Levels of Emotional Awareness Scale (Frewen, Lane, et al., 2008), higher levels of alexithymia (difficulties identifying and labeling emotional states; Edwards, 2022; Frewen, Dozois, Neufeld, & Lanius, 2008; Frewen, Lanius, et al., 2008; Yehuda et al., 1997), and intense levels of emotional numbing (feeling like they cannot experience emotions; Duek, Seidemann, Pietrzak, & Harpaz-Rotem, 2023; Frewen et al., 2012; Frewen & Lanius, 2006; Litz & Gray, 2002). As one traumatized individual eloquently described:

> "It's like a blank, I think about my kids and I feel nothing for them. I'll be sitting there feeling confused and numb, and I wonder what I'm supposed to be feeling. It's like dead space . . . and when that happens, I have trouble using words, finding my words, I can't talk."

Detaching from one's body through depersonalization is another way of escaping inner anguish. As explained in Chapter 4, the traumatized individual can feel as though they are looking down at their own body or as though their body is situated next to them. In more extreme cases, the person may feel as though their body no longer belongs to them. This dissociative strategy can be a brilliant way to dodge the excruciating agony associated with traumatic reexperiencing. As one traumatized person with depersonalization symptoms powerfully described:

> "For me, it was like a physical separation. Here's me up here in a tree, and here's this shell [body] down here [on the ground] that is being hurt and abused—but I can't feel it; I don't feel it; I am separate from that person; I am separate from my body now. My body is being hurt, but *I* am not being hurt. I think that is

one of the things that lets you survive because it is not *you*; you are not experiencing the full impact of what is happening. You are experiencing it, but *you* are not experiencing the full impact. The body is just a shell there that is being hurt. The vital part has left. It doesn't look like me—it looks like someone else is being hurt because me, I'm in the tree. Is there recognition of this shell? Yes, I would say there is some recognition. Is it *me*? I can't say that, 'yes, that was me' because I am in the tree, so I can't be down there."

Even though these out-of-body experiences helped this individual to survive the agony and dehumanization associated with their trauma, it left them feeling detached from the inner world of their sensations and feelings, thereby stripping them of their identity and their capacity to feel fully alive in the present.

I Feel, Therefore I Am: The War Within

The concept of conscious existence has been debated heavily in philosophy since the beginning of humankind. Dating back to 1637, René Descartes said the following: "Cogito, ergo sum," which translates to "I think; therefore I am," suggesting that thoughts are the basis of our emotions and existence. This quote has had a profound influence on society-at-large and has been the basis of many psychotherapeutic treatment modalities. It has led humans to feel comfortable relying principally on their ability to think via the reflective brain at the expense of valuing the mind, brain, and body connection. However, it is often forgotten that another philosopher, Baruch Spinoza, challenged Descartes's view 30 years later and proposed that the mind exists for the body's sake (Damasio, 2003). Spinoza argued that emotions stem from the body, and that bodily processes have a profound influence on how humans think and feel. For example, stress manifests in an array of physical symptoms, including ulcers, muscle tension and rigidity, irritable bowel syndrome, and shallow breathing. These bodily representations of mental stress can be considered foundational to how mental and bodily processes are intimately linked, where neglecting this relationship can preclude one's capacity to feel fully alive or to feel interconnected to other beings. The brain–gut connection is another crucial example to underscore the importance of attunement between mind and body. The gut flora has a critical influence on our mood and behavior to the extent of being labeled our "second brain." More than 350 years later, this debate still exists as therapists wrestle with how to weigh our thoughts and feelings with or without consideration of bodily processes (Barrett, 2017; Lindquist, Wager, Kober, Bliss-Moreau, & Barrett, 2012).

While the reflective brain defines humans' unique capacity to articulate thoughts and narratives, it reaches full maturation only at age 25; in contrast, the body fully develops much earlier within the context of an individual's relationship with a primary caregiver (Lebel, Walker, Leemans, Phillips, & Beaulieu, 2008).

As we discussed in Chapter 4, the attachment relationship, where the infant senses the soothing voice and touch of a caregiver, lays the foundation for one to feel inner sensations of safety and comfort (Siegel, 2020). These interoceptive sensations become baked into the infant's burgeoning sense of self, such that the self is comfortable with and deserving of positively valenced internal sensations. If one does not have the luxury of a secure, reliably loving attachment relationship, distressing and uncomfortable inner sensations may become the norm, and the ability to know what safety and comfort feels like at a visceral level can become severely compromised. This stunts the development of the foundation of human existence: to feel and be moved by emotion.

Humans are a mosaic of felt lived experiences—we use past feelings and visceral sensations to guide how we perceive our world. For example, seeing a child running to their father's arms may evoke strikingly different visceral sensations depending on past experience. For an individual who experienced a secure base and loving attachment, it may evoke a sensation of warmth in the chest as they are reminded of the unconditional love they received from their own father. Their narrative is that the world is a safe place, and that others are also experiencing the same love and connection that they felt as a child. By stark contrast, an individual like Tomas (see the case below), who experienced childhood sexual trauma after the sudden loss of his own father, sees the same interaction and feels a pit in his stomach. He associates this sensation with terror, self-disgust, anger, and grief. For Tomas, this fuels a narrative that the world is an unsafe place full of profound loneliness, where trust is not attainable and connection to others is dangerous. For yet another, this scene may evoke nothing at all. This flatness of sensory and emotional experience may create a profound sense of alienation from the self and others, where others seem to experience things completely unbeknownst to their own experience. A severely traumatized individual once said, "I don't know love. I have never experienced it. When I pet my cat, I wonder whether that's love, but I'm not sure." These examples clearly illustrate how different past experiences can shape and define our inner bodily sensations that directly influence the narratives and perceptions we derive from our world.

How the Past Shapes the Future

The brain, despite its small size in relation to the body, consumes a significant amount of our energy and accounts for 20% of the oxygen we breathe (Ndubuizu & LaManna, 2007). On a basic level, sensory input initiates neuronal communication through electrical signaling, which in turn guides behavior and attention. To maintain efficiency, our behavior and attention is guided to the most prominent stimulus experienced internally or externally. However, as described above, people can have vastly different reactions to the same stimulus (e.g., seeing a father playing with his child). To begin to understand this, we need to consider that the world and our perception of it is always changing. Because of the uncertainty of our external environment, we need to rely on past experiences to inform actions that make sense in our current surroundings. However, while we heavily rely on past experiences to guide behavior, we are never reacting within the same context because the parameters of our inner and outer environments are always changing. This leads to a constant updating of knowledge to optimally meet situational demands on a day-to-day basis, which is how we flexibly adapt and thrive in an ever-changing world while conserving the mind and body's energy.

After trauma, the malleability of the updating process diminishes as the body becomes conditioned to anticipate only threat. To minimize uncertainty, the individual always expects danger, thus losing the capacity to flexibly adapt to non-threatening situations. Brilliantly but devastatingly, the body adjusts to a new steady state of "under threat." The idea of "prepare for the worst, hope for the best" becomes "prepare for the worst and expect the worst." This existential shift causes many traumatized individuals to lose faith in themselves and the world, feeling deserving of only the worst possible outcomes in any situation. In cases of severe developmental trauma, this steady state of threat becomes imprinted from birth, robbing them of their basic right to feel safe in the world. These concepts are illustrated in the case examples below (deep brain reorienting [DBR] therapy discussed in the case is defined near the end of this chapter and explained further in Chapter 9).

CASE EXAMPLE: Tomas

Tomas is a resilient 62-year-old man who has suffered greatly since his childhood. Tomas grew up in France and moved to the United States with his parents and two siblings when he was 3 years old. The transition was very difficult for his parents. Both struggled with making ends meet, and Tomas's father had to work long hours to establish himself in the construction business. Tension in the family was high, and violence between Tomas's parents was a regular occurrence. Tragically, when Tomas was 5 years old, his father suddenly died from a heart attack. This left his mother feeling grief stricken and having to parent the children on her own. Furthermore, his mother had difficulty affording even the most basic groceries as the family faced poverty. Tomas's mother was therefore very grateful that she received support from her Catholic diocese, where the local priest regularly visited the family after Tomas's father's passing.

Tomas, the youngest child, had difficulty coping with the loss of his father and was yearning for a "replacement father." He was full of hope that the local priest from his church may be able to fulfill this role. Tomas always looked forward to the priest coming to the family's house and slowly began to confide in him. The priest began to invite Tomas to spend time with him at the rectory, making him feel special. As a result, Tomas sometimes felt jealous when seeing the priest give attention to other children. Nonetheless, Tomas was beginning to feel like his dream of having a "replacement father" was slowly coming true. During his visits to the rectory, Tomas would often cuddle with the priest, which made him feel loved and adored. Tomas trusted the priest more and more, and he felt that he could share some of his most closely held secrets with him.

After several months, the priest invited Tomas for a sleepover at his house. Tomas was thrilled and excited to be able to spend a longer period of intimate time with his newfound "father." Shortly after arriving at the priest's house, Tomas swam in the priest's pool and was playing water games with him. They went back into the house, where the priest invited Tomas to his bedroom to cuddle with him. Suddenly, things changed drastically. The priest's demeanor toward Tomas changed abruptly, and he became more demanding and assertive of his power. He insisted that Tomas lie on his side and implied that what was happening could not be discussed with others; otherwise, Tomas could lose his "specialness" and his intimate relationship with the priest. Tomas was utterly confused and could not comprehend what was happening. He remembers the priest beginning to anally rape him to the point where Tomas zoned out and disconnected from his body (depersonalization), as well as from the reality around him (derealization). Tomas later came to and tried to escape from the house. Unfortunately, it was dark, and he was not able to find his way home. In desperation, he found an axe to help defend himself against the priest but realized he could not overpower him. He therefore placed the axe beside the bed and spent the rest of the night in terror alongside the priest. From that day forward, things changed for Tomas.

The priest slowly started to withdraw from Tomas. Every time Tomas became close to another person, he now became filled with rage, self-disgust, and mistrust. The feelings of love and trust he had developed for the priest were now coupled with the violence he had experienced by him, and feelings of rage, self-disgust, and mistrust now permeated every relationship throughout his childhood and adult life. Indeed, Tomas has never been able to sustain a relationship for longer than 1 year. Every time Tomas has felt any semblance of closeness or sexual arousal, he flashes back to the feelings associated with the anal rape. The tragic aftermath of what was one of the most intimate relationships he ever had left Tomas feeling devastated and undeserving of love or social connection, even from his mother. He was left feeling deserted, abandoned, and exiled.

Tomas has been in therapy for most of his life to come to terms with this life-shattering event. He has received treatment using multiple modalities, including cognitive processing therapy, dialectical behavior therapy, EMDR, internal family systems, neurofeedback, and psychedelic-assisted psychotherapy, which have prevented him from committing suicide and helped him to cope over the years. However, it was not until he received DBR therapy, which involves attending to tension in the head and neck muscles while processing traumatic shock and visceral emotion, that he slowly started to be able to uncouple feelings of closeness, love, and sexual arousal from rage, self-disgust, and mistrust. Tomas is continuing to process these difficult emotions and now feels less hijacked by them when navigating an intimate relationship. For the first time, he has hope that he will be able to maintain a trusting relationship sometime before the end of his life.

Developing Behavioral Habits to Foster Survival after Trauma: How Safety Becomes Uncertainty

How do traumatized individuals adapt to grossly unpredictable environments involving chronic inescapable threat in order to maintain their own survival? Active inference (Friston, Kilner, & Harrison, 2006; Friston, Mattout, & Kilner, 2011) proposes an answer to this question. In this context, this theory postulates that the brain is constantly generating predictions about what sensory input it expects to receive based on learning and experience. In other words, past experiences form internal models of sensory expectation, which are constantly updated to minimize the discrepancy between predictions and sensory input. This process, known as prediction error, ultimately helps the system become more efficient and reduces the burden or stress that comes with unpredictability and uncertainty. This is the body's way to maintain a steady state unique to the individual, where *allostasis* (i.e., a physiological process that promotes internal balance) facilitates a state of balance among all body systems needed for the brain, mind, and body to survive and function optimally.

When faced with a familiar situation, we feel an urge to react similarly based on knowledge from previous experience in order to conserve energy and reduce stress, akin to when we discussed sensory imprints in Chapter 3. The more consistent the sensory experience is, the more habitual the action becomes. This habituation is facilitated by a brain structure in the emotional learning brain called the striatum, which can receive input from the survival brain to initiate habitual movements without conscious planning at the level of the reflective brain. For example, a skilled piano player exhibits habitual motor patterns that are extremely precise while navigating a complex Rachmaninoff concerto. The hands are further propelled by the raw emotion experienced, allowing the musician to play with emotion and vigor. Repeated practicing of the concerto then forms the long-term belief that they possess competence and mastery over the piece. In Tomas's case, seeing the priest prior to the rape habitually evoked visceral bodily sensations of warmth and joy. Over time, this habitual experience had a profound effect on his belief system, such that the priest was a safe and nurturing figure in his life (see Figure 6.1). These repeated visceral feelings of warmth and safety led him to continue approaching the priest which, in turn, fostered long-term beliefs that the priest and the world were safe and could be fully trusted.

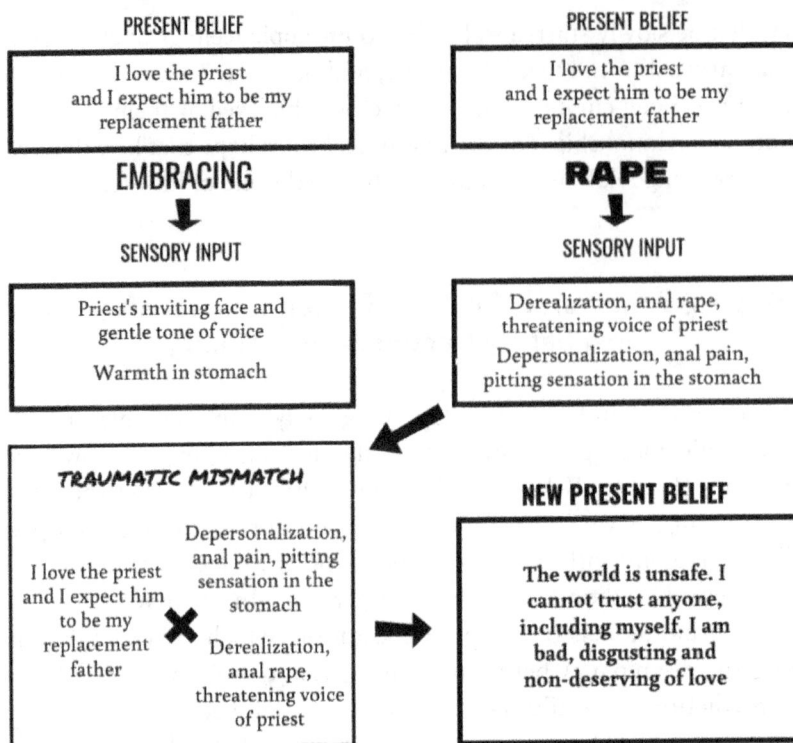

FIGURE 6.1. Updating beliefs after trauma through the lens of prediction errors.

However, if the degree of unpredictability or uncertainty of a situation increases, it may require more conscious planning at the level of the reflective brain to adapt to the new situation. If the musician starts practicing the Rachmaninoff concerto on the plastic keys of a keyboard instead of the wooden keys of a grand piano, the sensory feedback differs significantly and alters the raw emotion elicited while performing; this necessitates that the reflective brain override the habitual actions. Elicitation of the reflective brain facilitates the conscious updating of hand movements when playing the keyboard. For Tomas, the habitual visceral bodily sensations of joy and warmth prior to the rape created an urge to run toward the priest and hug him. However, if he saw the priest interacting with other boys, it would evoke a pit sensation in his stomach reminiscent of rage and jealousy over the priest's inaccessibility, causing him to refrain from approaching the priest (Figure 6.1). The concept of active inference can also be applied to racial trauma, where racialized communities have learned to expect danger and discrimination in their everyday lives (Bryant-Davis, 2007; Bryant-Davis, Chung, & Tillman, 2009; Elbasheir et al., 2024; Fani et al., 2021; Fani, Fulton, & Botzanowski, 2024). This is illustrated in the following case example that was contributed by two Black, Indigenous, or people of color therapists who work in the field of racial trauma in the United States.

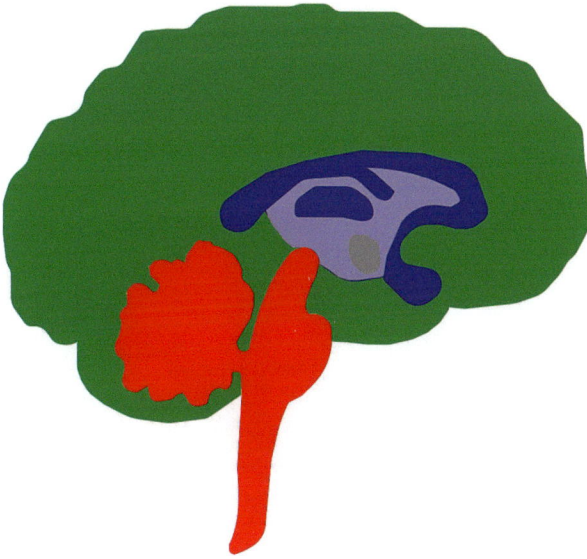

PLATE 1.1. The three sections of the brain, including the survival brain (red), emotional learning brain (blue), and the reflective brain (green).

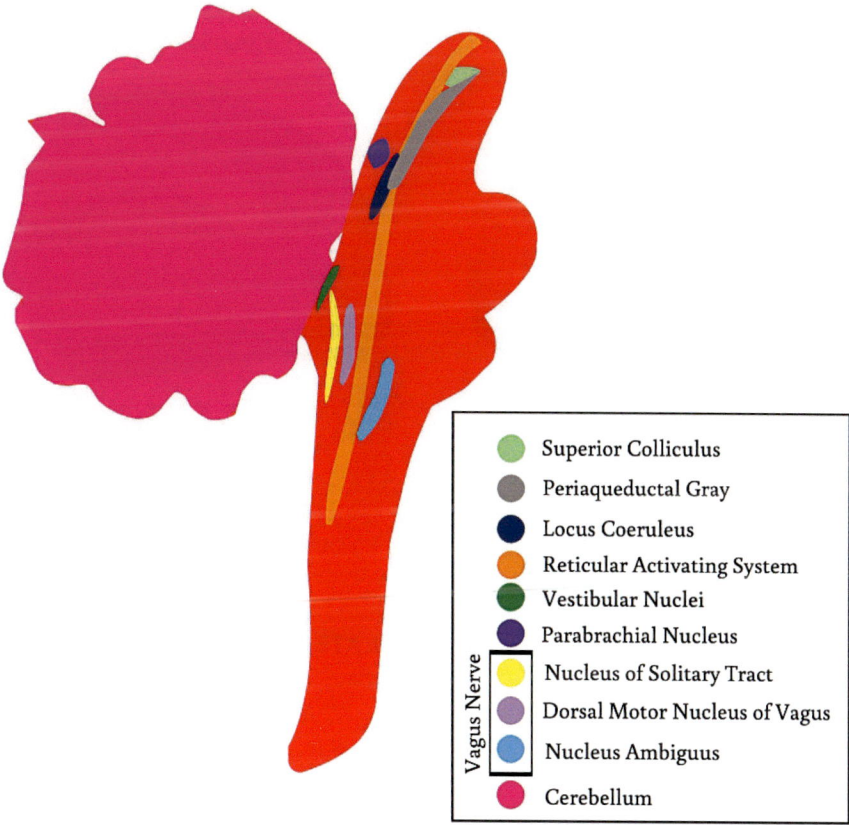

Superior Colliculus
Periaqueductal Gray
Locus Coeruleus
Reticular Activating System
Vestibular Nuclei
Parabrachial Nucleus
Nucleus of Solitary Tract
Dorsal Motor Nucleus of Vagus
Nucleus Ambiguus
Cerebellum

Vagus Nerve

PLATE 1.2. The survival brain.

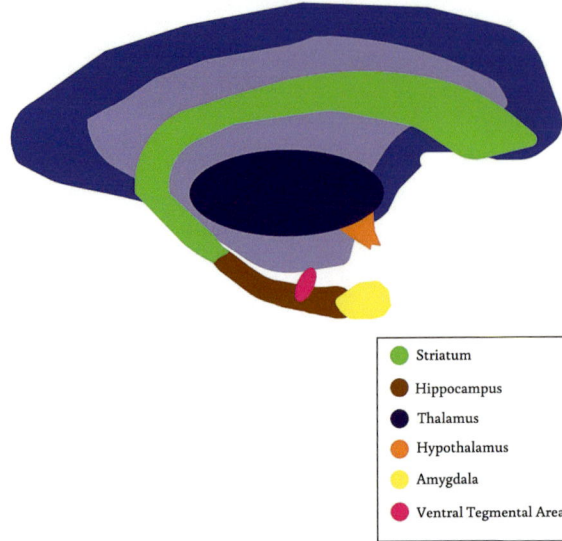

PLATE 1.3. The emotional learning brain.

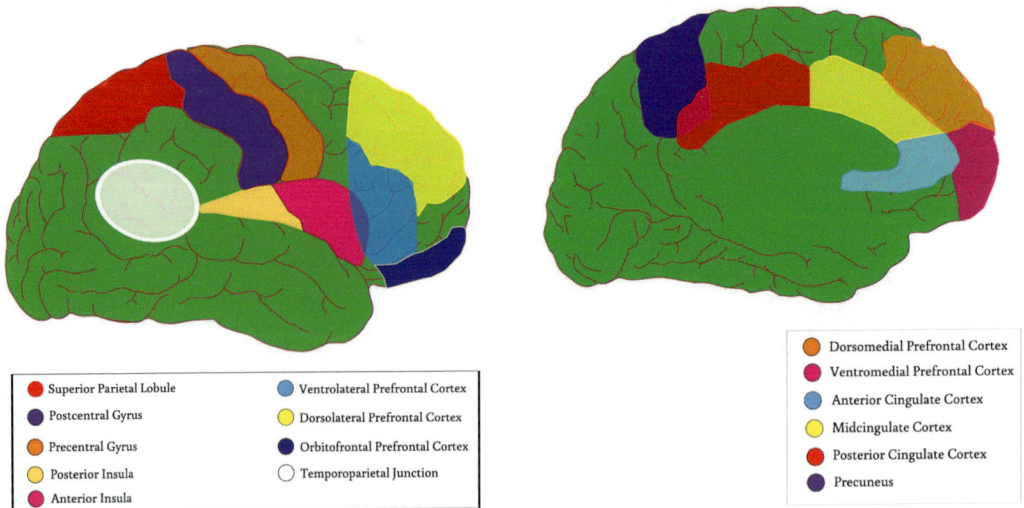

Striatum
Hippocampus
Thalamus
Hypothalamus
Amygdala
Ventral Tegmental Area

PLATE 1.4A. The reflective brain: lateral view.

Superior Parietal Lobule
Postcentral Gyrus
Precentral Gyrus
Posterior Insula
Anterior Insula
Ventrolateral Prefrontal Cortex
Dorsolateral Prefrontal Cortex
Orbitofrontal Prefrontal Cortex
Temporoparietal Junction

PLATE 1.4B. The reflective brain: medial view.

Dorsomedial Prefrontal Cortex
Ventromedial Prefrontal Cortex
Anterior Cingulate Cortex
Midcingulate Cortex
Posterior Cingulate Cortex
Precuneus

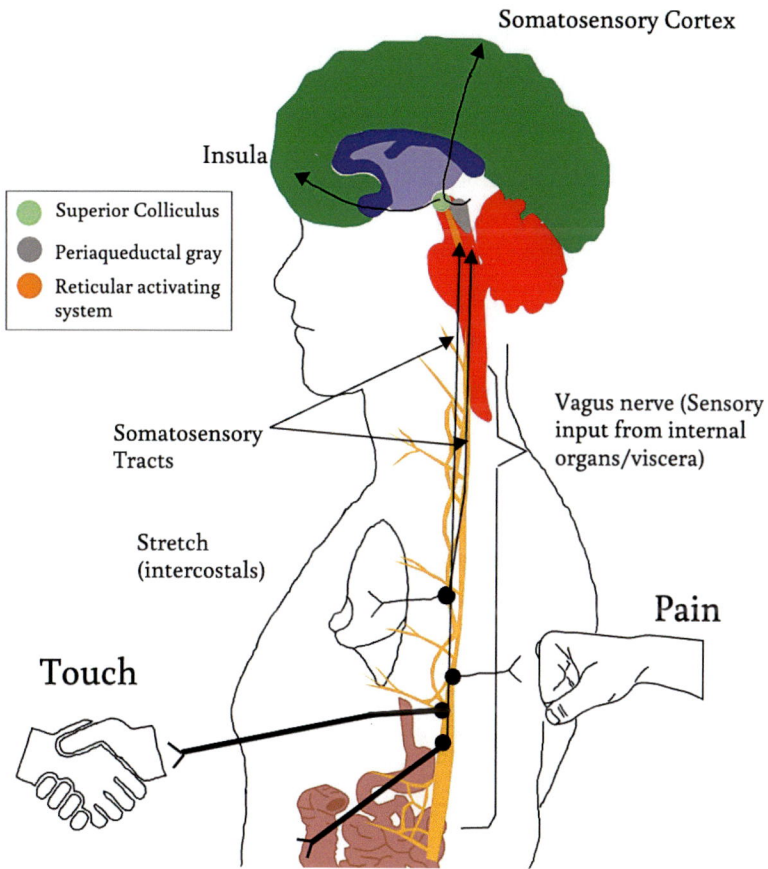

PLATE 2.1. Somatosensory pathways to the brain.

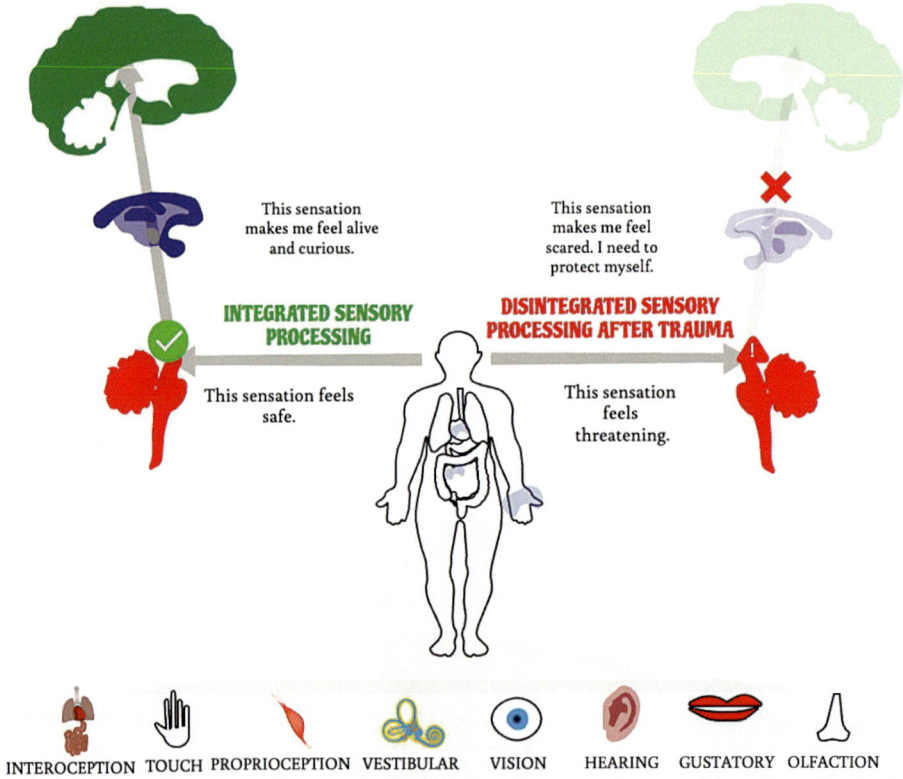

I can recognize this sensation as pleasant.
I am not afraid to feel it again.

This is terrifying. My faster survival and
emotional learning brain have taken over.

This sensation
makes me feel alive
and curious.

This sensation
makes me feel
scared. I need to
protect myself.

INTEGRATED SENSORY
PROCESSING

DISINTEGRATED SENSORY
PROCESSING AFTER TRAUMA

This sensation feels
safe.

This sensation
feels
threatening.

INTEROCEPTION TOUCH PROPRIOCEPTION VESTIBULAR VISION HEARING GUSTATORY OLFACTION

PLATE 3.1. Sensory integration versus sensory disintegration after trauma.

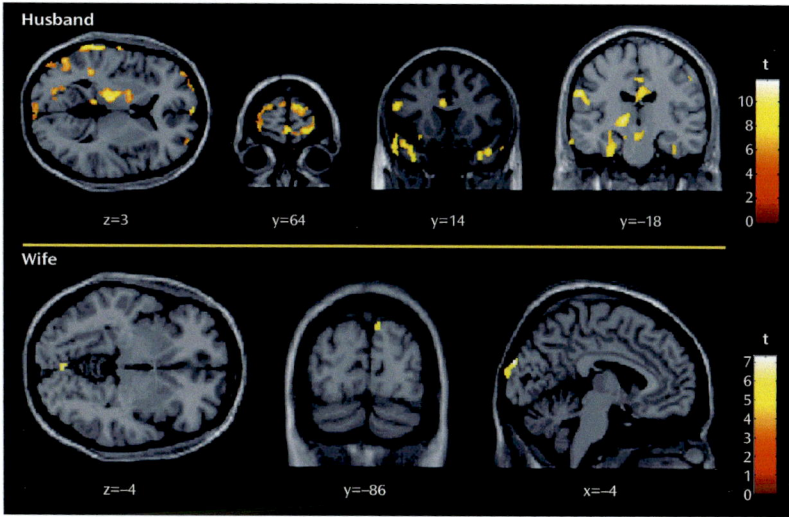

PLATE 4.1. (A) fMRI of the husband's brain upon traumatic memory recall of the car accident; (B) fMRI of the wife's brain upon traumatic memory recall of the same car accident. From Lanius et al. (2003).

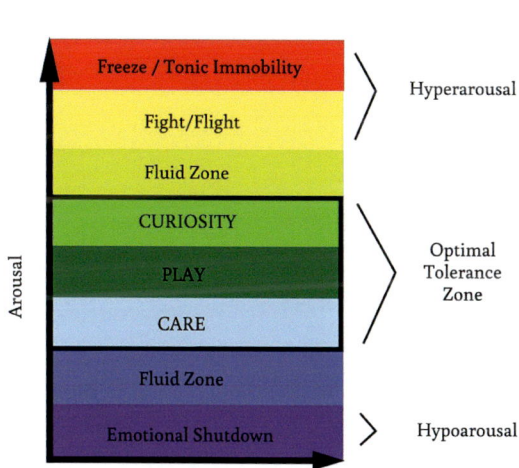

PLATE 4.2. A depiction of the window of tolerance. Based on Siegel (1999) and Warner et al. (2020).

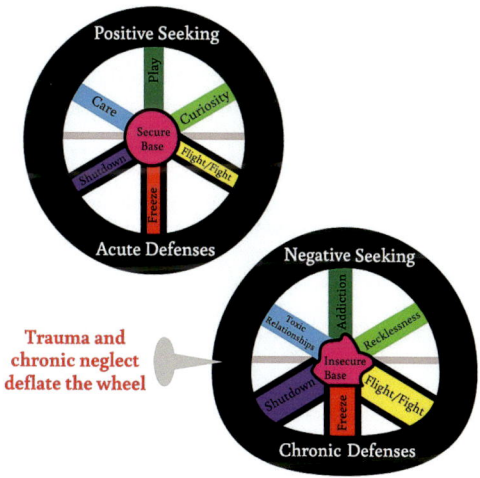

PLATE 4.3. The wheel of discovery. Here, positive seeking is associated with a secure attachment. In contrast, negative seeking can be associated with an insecure attachment and chronic defensive responses that can dampen curiosity, care, and play, thus impeding movement forward in life and the therapeutic setting.

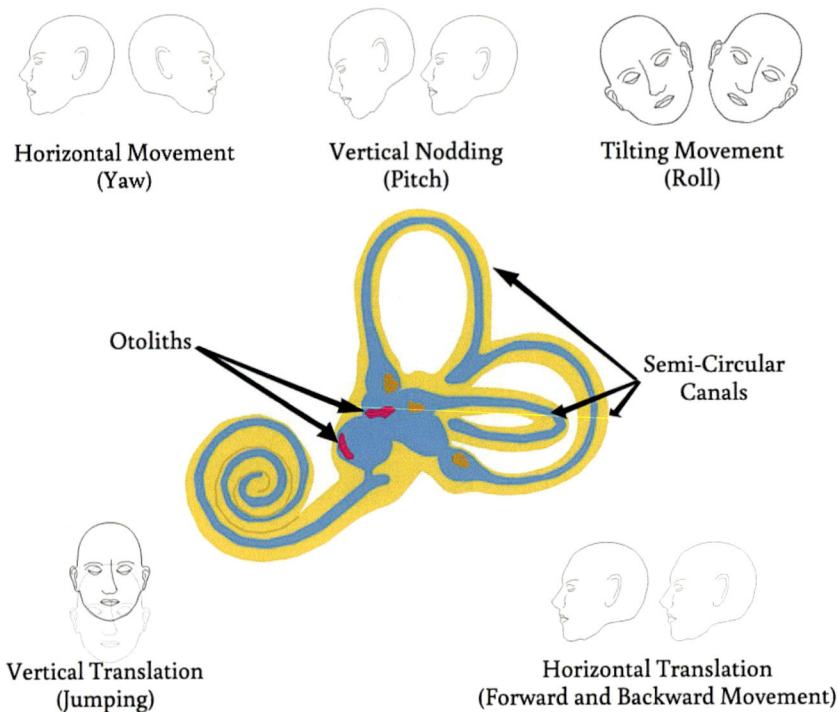

Horizontal Movement
(Yaw)

Vertical Nodding
(Pitch)

Tilting Movement
(Roll)

Otoliths

Semi-Circular
Canals

Vertical Translation
(Jumping)

Horizontal Translation
(Forward and Backward Movement)

PLATE 5.1. Vestibular organs and the head movements they detect.

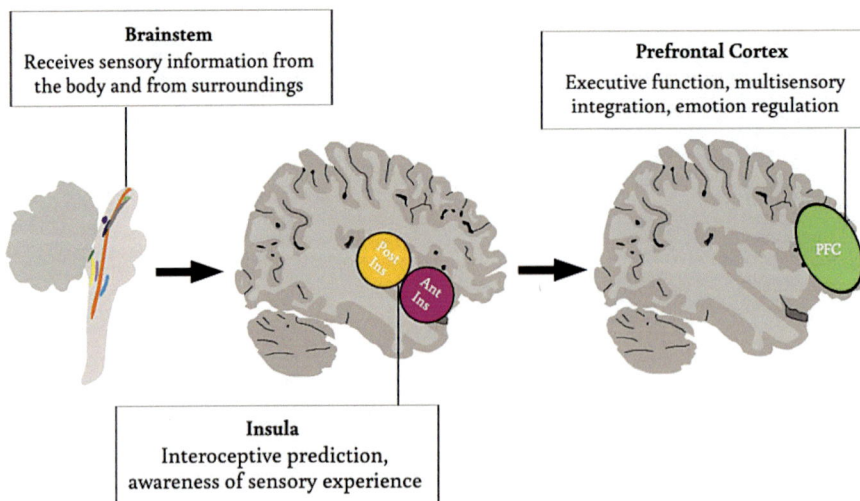

Brainstem
Receives sensory information from
the body and from surroundings

Prefrontal Cortex
Executive function, multisensory
integration, emotion regulation

Post
Ins

Ant
Ins

PFC

Insula
Interoceptive prediction,
awareness of sensory experience

PLATE 6.1. Typical chain of sensory transmission in the brain. Abbreviations: Post Ins = posterior insula; Ant Ins = anterior insula; PFC = prefrontal cortex.

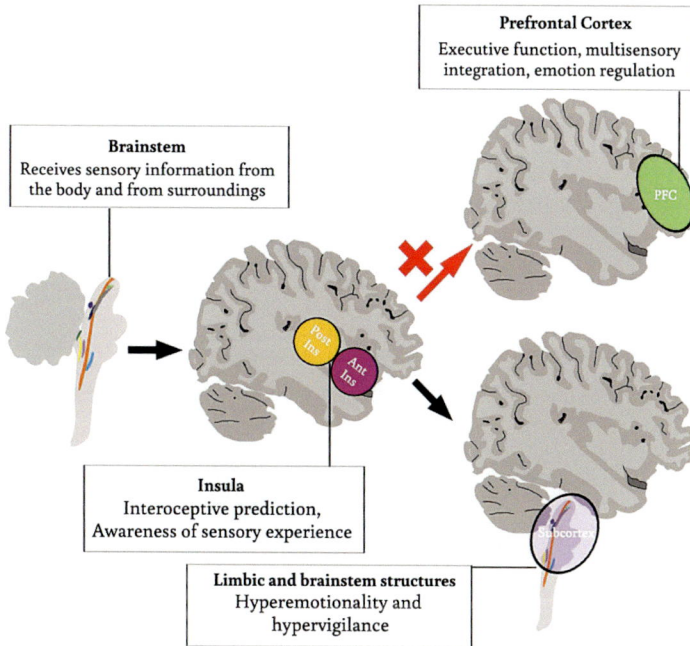

PLATE 6.2. Chain of sensory transmission in the brain among individuals with PTSD. Instead of sensory information traveling to the prefrontal cortex for higher-order processing, it is redirected to subcortical structures in the innate alarm system. Abbreviations: Post Ins = posterior insula; Ant Ins = anterior insula; PFC = prefrontal cortex.

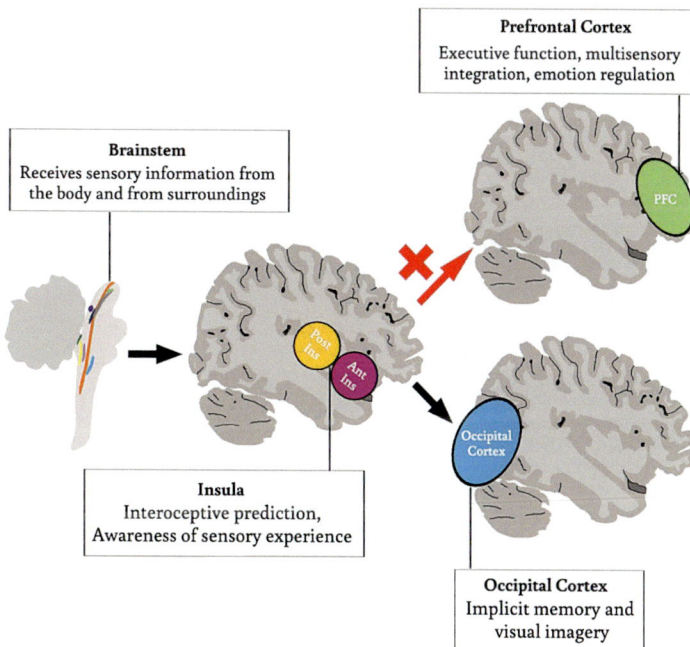

PLATE 6.3. Chain of sensory transmission in the brain among individuals with the PTSD dissociative subtype. Instead of sensory information traveling to the prefrontal cortex for higher-order processing, it is redirected to the occipital cortex. Abbreviations: Post Ins = posterior insula; Ant Ins = anterior insula; PFC = prefrontal cortex.

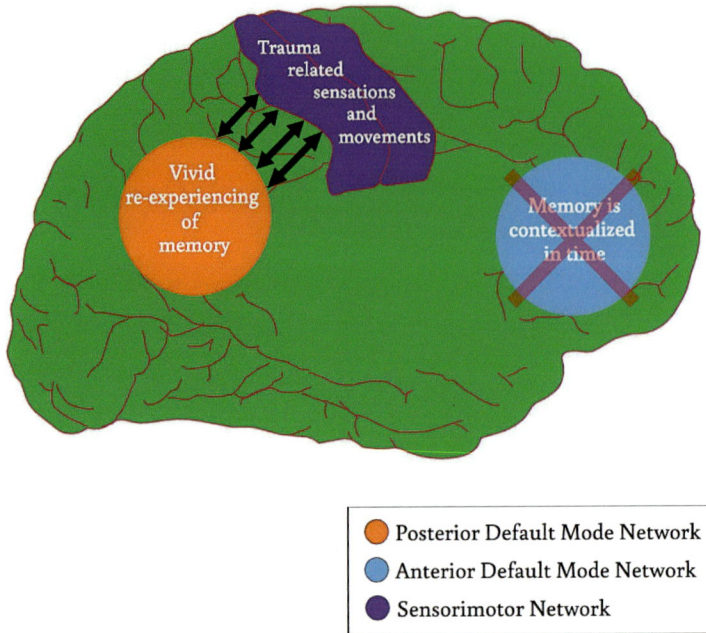

PLATE 8.1. Reliving is not remembering. How the default mode network interacts with the sensorimotor network to create reliving experiences among traumatized individuals.

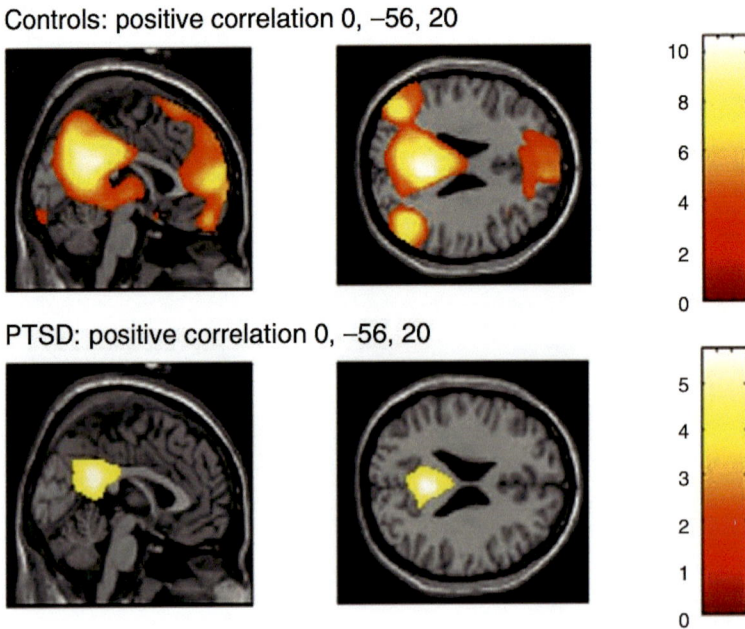

PLATE 8.2. Default mode network in PTSD versus healthy controls. From Bluhm et al. (2009, Fig. 1).

CASE EXAMPLE: The Traffic Stop

By Debra Chatman-Finley, LPC, NCC, and Gliceria Pérez, LCSW

In June 2019, we were driving home from a Soul Work Conference for "Therapists of Color and Their White Allies" in Connecticut. We felt safe there and were euphoric and energized. It was a great conference weekend filled with colleagues, stories, music, dancing, food, and excellent presenters. We were enjoying the ride home until we saw a New Jersey state trooper stare at us as we drove by him. After a few minutes, Debra, who was driving, said, "He's following us, and I think he's going to pull us over." Our hearts began to race.

We weren't speeding but a minute or so later, as we approached our exit from the highway, Debra properly signaled and took the exit ramp to the street that led to Debra's house. It was then we saw his flashing lights and we pulled over. After we pulled over and before the officer came to the car, Gliceria said in hushed tones, "Debra, put your hands on the dashboard." She was already facing forward with her hands on the dashboard. Her voice echoed concern bordering on fear.

When the trooper, a White male, exited his car, instead of coming to the driver's side of our car where Debra was, he suddenly appeared on the passenger side with his hands on his gun and told Gliceria to roll down the window. He peered into the car and said, "Do you know why I pulled you over?"

Debra said "no." To which he replied, "You were driving while on your cell phone." Debra told him that she was not using her cell phone because it was in her purse in the back seat, and he must have mistaken her sunglasses for a cell phone.

The state trooper never took his hand off his gun as he asked for Debra's license, registration, and insurance. He then walked back to his car to check her information and at this point Debra put her hands on the dashboard and kept them there. When he came back to the car his hand was still on his gun and he said, "Okay, this time I'm going to let you go." He made it sound like he was doing us a favor, even though we had done nothing wrong and should never have been pulled over in the first place. Nonetheless, we thanked him and said nothing else.

That should have been the end of our encounter, but it was not. We drove off and continued the drive to Debra's home. We then noticed that the trooper was still following us but no longer had on his flashing red lights.

We were scared and so many thoughts raced through our minds in a matter of seconds. They were all thoughts of being Black and Latina and how he would get away with killing us. He followed us to Debra's home and then he finally drove away. It was over but it really was not over. By the time we got into Debra's house, we were both shaking, and her husband asked if we had taken down his badge number or name. Sadly, we never thought about it in the moment, and even if we had, we were too frightened to do so.

We kept replaying and talking about the incident, especially how he kept his hand on his gun and then followed us all the way home after the initial stop. Why? What was he thinking? What did we do to make him follow us other than be two women of color? Did he think we stole the car? Was he hoping to catch us committing a crime, so he could justifiably shoot us?

Although we were home, it was still hard to feel safe. The entire incident left us feeling afraid. The backdrop for our fear was not only the attitude and unwarranted intimidation by the police officer keeping his hand on his gun during the entire incident but it was also the growing frequency of police killing unarmed Black people in the years leading up to our traffic stop, including Eric Garner, Michael Brown, and a 12-year-old boy, Tamir Rice, just to name a few. Even though Sandra Bland was not shot and killed, she died in a holding cell after an unwarranted traffic stop led to her arrest for not being "cooperative."

Shortly after our traffic stop by the police, the deaths of unarmed Black people seemed to increase in frequency with the deaths of Philando Castile, Breonna Taylor, and the out-and-out murder of George Floyd adding to our feelings of insecurity and fear.

The incident remains with us to this day whenever we see a state trooper or any police officer or whenever we see on the news that there was another unwarranted killing of a person of color. Being two people of color, the continued killing of unarmed Black people by the police adds to our continued feeling of insecurity, fear, and sadness coupled with a deep breath of relief that we were not added to the toll.

Finding a New Steady State after Trauma: Where Unpredictability Becomes Survival

In the aftermath of trauma, the body's steady state of anticipating and orienting toward threat can be difficult to emerge from because danger is viewed as an inevitability. If the theory of active inference postulates that the body is always striving to conserve energy and maintain a state of physiological equilibrium, we expect that the brain and body will avoid uncertainty and refrain from disrupting the body's steady state. However, in the aftermath of trauma, one's experience of their inner world and overarching belief systems drastically shift such that they consistently experience the world as an unsafe, uncertain, and unpredictable place in which they do not belong. This causes individuals to be chronically hypervigilant of their surroundings (see discussion about the defense cascade model in Chapter 4), where safety and relaxation can be perceived as vulnerable and dangerous. Hence, entering a state of relaxation would require less vigilance and more "letting go," which a traumatized individual may couple with a loss of safety, as it makes them feel vulnerable to further insults. In turn, hypervigilance eventually becomes the body's new steady state, and the only state in which the individual feels some level of familiarity. Among severely traumatized individuals, extreme levels of hypervigilance can deplete the energy requirements to sustain this state, leading to a psychological escape through dissociation.

Active inference helps us to conceptualize why traumatized individuals find themselves pulled toward unsafe environments and relationships. In the case of Tomas, after he was raped, he embodied a chronic state of hypervigilance in any situation where love and intimacy could arise that manifested as rage, self-disgust, and mistrust. These feelings felt familiar; it requires less energy to respond with familiar patterns than to expend energy and respond differently. The tradeoff was a profound detachment and disconnection from others, including his own mother, resulting in an instinctual avoidance of romantic partnerships. In other cases, traumatized individuals subconsciously seek out dangerous or fear-inducing situations that maintain a steady state of chronic hypervigilance, such as abusive relationships or chaotically demanding work environments. This gravitation toward danger coincides with sensations and long-term belief systems that the world and others are untrustworthy and unsafe. Here, they are further predisposed to a cycle of repetition compulsion of past traumas, where the individual perpetually reexperiences the familiar horrors. This is known as *repetition compulsion*, the loop that entangles many traumatized individuals, causing them to repeat past traumas (Herman, 1992a, 2015; van der Kolk, 1989).

Among children who experienced repeated abuse, this predisposition to unsafe situations may be the only reality they know. There was never a safe place to find refuge. Even if there were access to safety, they may not have been able to embrace it fully beneath the persistently looming threat of danger. Hence, this predisposition can exacerbate their vulnerability to further psychological insult and even lead to a subconscious need to reenact early traumas. For example, if a child grew up in a physically and/or sexually abusive environment, they may be susceptible to entering abusive adult relationships (Briere, Runtz, & Rodd, 2024). This can be especially prominent in cases where individuals have endured prolonged and repeated trauma, where social conditions can breed subordination and powerlessness among victims.

Critically, repeated acts of violence are not necessary to sustain these social conditions; a single act of violence can serve to instill prolonged fear among victims. Judith Herman (1992a) described this as part of a grooming response from perpetrators, where they exert coercive control to sustain a steady state of submission from victims and use violence as the most extreme method of enforcing submission to one's will. This is further discussed in Chapter 8. Individuals who have experienced unpredictable caregiving environments during childhood can be more vulnerable to grooming, as they may readily regress to a familiar state of unpredictability and chaos. These perpetrators can even exert coercive control over their victims' bodily functions, affecting one's interoceptive sense at a deep visceral level and conditioning a steady state of disequilibrium in the body. For example, withholding food (e.g., giving it only as a reward), making individuals soil themselves, and controlling sleep claims a sense of ownership over the victim's living body and robs them of their own senses of interoception and agency. This creates a profound sense of helplessness in the victim and engenders firm beliefs that the world is a hopeless and dangerous place where they cannot effect change. They end up feeling exiled and discarded. Lacking a sense of body ownership may also foster *kinesthetic anesthesia*, which refers to a visceral sense that one's own body disappears. Of course, this leads to great losses of agency and of self where the traumatized individual becomes a passive bystander in their own life. Life becomes a meaningless series of mechanical motions devoid of purpose or feeling.

Paving the Way to Welcoming One's Inner Sensations after Trauma

The immense emotional toll of traumatic events often leaves individuals overwhelmed and consumed by clinical symptoms that have negative cascading impacts on higher-order structures in the reflective brain—namely, the prefrontal cortex, which is essential for introspection and emotion regulation. Specifically, the prefrontal cortex enables us to carry out abstract reasoning, a process that inherently distances us from past events and helps to develop rational thoughts about them that are less emotionally charged. This thereby facilitates the processing and integration of traumatic memories, which are essential processes for healing. Research into the neurobiology of PTSD has repeatedly demonstrated that its clinical profile is directly linked to altered levels of activation at the level of the prefrontal cortex (Bluhm et al., 2009; Fenster, Lebois, Ressler, & Suh, 2018; Harricharan et al., 2019; Lanius, Terpou, & McKinnon, 2020; Lanius et al., 2010), which may manifest as persistent feelings of unsafety despite the absence of threat. The inability of the prefrontal cortex to engage abstract reasoning and provide context to situations and sensory input may lead to irrationally high levels of vigilance, extreme fatigue from emotional expenditure related to traumatic reminders, feelings of negative self-worth (e.g., shame, guilt), and disembodied emotional detachment from inner emotional turmoil. The prefrontal cortex serves as a hub for most neural networks in the brain and its dysfunction can severely limit one's capacity for everyday functioning.

Additional reflective brain structures that are critical for interoceptive awareness (understanding inner bodily sensations) and identifying emotion are affected after trauma. As discussed earlier in this chapter, the insula is involved in the neural transmission of inner interoceptive sensations, relaying sensory information from the survival and emotional learning brains to the prefrontal cortex in

the reflective brain (see Plate 6.1). Here, the insula creates an interoceptive inference, where interoceptive signals that carry information about our internal visceral states (e.g., pain, temperature) are weighed against predictive models that
help detect why these signals occur. Critically, Harricharan and colleagues (2019)
found that, at rest, individuals with PTSD demonstrated starkly different functional connections between the insula and other structures in the brain when
compared to healthy controls (see Plate 6.2). The study showed that healthy controls demonstrated greater insula functional connectivity with the dorsolateral
prefrontal cortex when compared to traumatized individuals. Conversely, individuals with PTSD and its dissociative subtype as compared to healthy controls
showed greater insula functional connectivity with structures in the survival and
emotional learning brains (e.g., periaqueductal gray, amygdala) and the occipital
cortex, respectively (see Plate 6.3). Among individuals with PTSD, this increased
insula connectivity with structures in the lower brain layers suggests that it plays
a role in maintaining symptoms related to feeling unsafe and dysregulated arousal
(e.g., hypervigilance). Interestingly, it is hypothesized that those with the PTSD
dissociative subtype may initiate compensatory brain pathways in posterior brain
structures (e.g., occipital lobe) to account for deficits experienced at the level of
the prefrontal cortex. As we saw in Chapter 5, individuals with both types of
PTSD also experience difficulty registering vestibular information, also leading
to hypervigilance.

Currently, many of the existing first-line treatments for PTSD rely heavily on access to the reflective brain, given their reliance on verbal language and
self-reflection on one's own behaviors. In other words, they *start* by challenging
core beliefs and applying complex reasoning to aid in the processing of traumatic
memories, which are functions primarily facilitated by the prefrontal cortex in the
reflective brain. However, if the prefrontal cortex is operating at a limited capacity, it hinders the ability to reap the full benefit of these treatments. Consequently,
traumatized individuals may be left feeling inadequate or hopeless in their respective healing journeys if they are initially unable to engage in these treatments—in
some cases, this sense of failure may further exacerbate their symptoms. This
points to an urgent need to develop brain-guided treatments that target an alternative entry point at a lower level of the brain that can be more easily accessed. It
may therefore be helpful to first incorporate adjunctive therapeutic strategies that
target structures in the survival and emotional learning brains that are involved
in understanding the raw visceral sensations experienced in the body. Here, an
emphasis on encouraging individuals to gradually experience and tolerate deep visceral sensations related to their inner emotional turmoil through adjunctive strategies discussed below can promote interoceptive awareness and begin to reengage
the prefrontal cortex slowly through neuroplasticity.

Fostering awareness and tolerance of the raw visceral sensations propagated
from within the body may therefore be a crucial first step in understanding how

and why the individual experiences, interprets, and labels emotions in distressing ways in the aftermath of trauma. Critically, building this awareness involves utilizing the parts of the brain that *are* online among these individuals, especially the survival brain's connections to the insula for the integration of interoception and somatosensation (i.e., touch and proprioception), the senses that allow us to *feel*. The incorporation of sensory-based strategies and/or adjunctive application of bottom-up therapies may enhance and optimize mainstream treatments by inspiring a bridge between knowing one's raw bodily sensations (visceral pain or fluttering, hollowing in the heart space) and their reflective, higher self-related thoughts ("I am worthless," "I am broken"). We hypothesize that propagating interoceptive experiences at the level of the insula can help to link the lower-brain structures in the survival and emotional learning brains with the prefrontal cortex in the higher reflective brain (Foa & Rothbaum, 1998; Fosha, 2002; Greenberg & Goldman, 2019; Thomaes et al., 2014), the latter being a primary target for trauma-focused treatments in changing thoughts and beliefs (Beck, 2021; Resick, Monson, & Chard, 2017). For example, Fonzo and colleagues (2017) showed that following prolonged exposure therapy, the anterior insula moderated activation of the dorsolateral prefrontal cortex during processing of fearful emotional stimuli. Moreover, consistent with Kluetsch and colleagues (2014) and Nicholson and associates (2020), Fonzo et al. showed that insular activity following neurofeedback was linked to restoration of dorsomedial prefrontal cortex activity, a pivotal brain structure for introspection and self-reflection.

As we have outlined in this chapter, there is a great need to consider the visceral sensations and affect (raw emotion) underlying the distressing and sometimes unmanageable emotional responses to trauma-relevant stimuli experienced by traumatized individuals. Various forms of practices, exercises, and targeted treatment approaches directly address these raw internal sensations, which can collectively be called "interoceptive-based interventions." Interoceptive-based interventions have been defined as those that promote and explicitly encourage self-reflection upon internal bodily states or experiences (Heim et al., 2023). These interventions can range anywhere from traditional Eastern practices of yoga and meditation to integrative exercise programs. Some examples include the following, which all aim to cultivate a safe connection between the internal world and the brain in the context of the external environment, which in turn, may facilitate a sense of belonging and trust within the body and the world:

- Mindfulness meditation
- Body scans (slow, progressive attention to each part of the body, including the internal state)
- Progressive muscle relaxation (gradually tensing and then relaxing each muscle group in the body)
- Guided awareness of bodily responses to physical exercise (e.g., heart rate, temperature increases)

- Interoceptive aspects of sensorimotor/somatic experiencing-based psychotherapy (becoming mindful of and observing bodily signals as a facet of treatment)
- DBR (attending to tension in head and neck muscles while processing traumatic shock and visceral emotion)

Despite the heterogeneity of interoceptive-based approaches, they all share a fundamental principle: improving the capacity to tolerate and accept one's internal state can lead to improvements in posttraumatic symptoms. Specifically, those who can notice and better tolerate their internal sensations may experience decreased avoidance of and lessened reactivity to reminders of past traumas. Ultimately, building trust in one's ability to effectively navigate the undulating waves of raw visceral sensations by way of anchoring and orienting the body's interoceptive world in the present moment can foster an improved balance between their internal and external sensory worlds (see Bridging to Practice 6 for additional guidance about how to implement this in a therapeutic setting).

Importantly, research has found that symptom improvements are stronger when they target both bottom-up (awareness of internal sensations) *and* top-down (thoughts and beliefs about internal sensations) dimensions of interoception (Heim et al., 2023). Examples of such treatments can include but are not limited to the following:

- Sensory-based expressive arts therapy (Malchiodi, 2022)
- Electroencephalogram (EEG) neurofeedback (Fisher, 2014; Nicholson et al., 2020)
- Equine-assisted psychotherapy (Mueller & McCullough, 2017; Naste et al., 2018; Palomar-Ciria & Bello, 2023)
- Strategies that target autonomic awareness (Dana, 2018)
- Transcutaneous vagal nerve stimulation (Lamb, Porges, Lewis, & Williamson, 2017)

Taken together, these findings support the utilization of bidirectional treatment approaches that integrate raw visceral sensations with cognitive appraisal.

BRIDGING TO PRACTICE 6

**Learning to Reinhabit the Body:
Bringing Interoceptive Awareness Online**

As discussed in the chapter, developing an individual's interoceptive awareness sets up a critical foundation for treatment, where teaching an individual to attend to sensations of their inner body can facilitate body ownership and help make sense of their feelings. It can be difficult to identify inner sensations in the body, especially if a client is particularly numb or avoidant of their emotions and/or prone to experiencing feelings of disembodiment.

Part A: Developing a Sense of Our Body

For clients who feel severely disconnected from their bodies, you can try offering various forms of exteroceptive sensory input, such as ice cubes, weighted blankets, tuning forks, an exercise ball, or self-applied pressure on a body part of their choice. Here, you can have the client choose the amount, intensity, and duration of the pressure. Furthermore, this can also involve encouraging the client to change between different posture positions (e.g., moving from a head-down, sunken shoulders position to an upright forward-facing position and reflecting on changes to the inner sensations with the client). Be aware that this process can take weeks to months among clients who are severely disconnected from their bodies (refer to Bridging to Practice features in Chapters 2, 3, and 5). It is imperative to spend time developing this foundational layer of interoceptive awareness to maximize the client's potential.

Part B: Connecting Bodily Sensations to Feelings and Emotions

It may take time for clients to find words that articulate these sensations let alone identify the emotions that underpin them. Here, it is imperative to start developing an individual's internal sense of the body step-by-step in a titrated manner, identifying the location of an inner visceral sensation and encouraging them to explore it with curiosity. The therapist can start by encouraging their client to explore any current bodily sensation they are experiencing during the session to help teach the individual to attend to sensations of their inner body. Rather than having them find words, the therapist can use a blank body map (refer to Bridging to Practice 1 in Chapter 1) and ask the client to identify *where* in the body they are feeling the inner bodily sensation. The individual can shade in the area of the body where they feel the sensation and even use colors, such as red and blue, to indicate if the sensation feels "hot" (red) or "cold" (blue). Have the client increasingly sit with this sensation at a gradual pace, whether it is 1 second, then 2 seconds, 5 seconds, and so on.

Over time, encourage the individual to focus on that sensation in the particular area of the body and see if they can find any basic words to describe it. For example, if an individual feels a "cold sensation in the stomach," they may be able to identify it further as "It feels cold, almost like it's sinking into a pit in my stomach." From here, they may be able to identify some basic form of raw emotion connected to the sensation, like "fear," "rage," or "panic," based on Panksepp's (1998) description of raw emotions identified in primary-process consciousness in the survival and emotional learning brain layers (see potential list of raw emotions below). To build on this, the client may be able to connect the sensation to higher-order emotions like sadness, shame, guilt, or anger, using the reflective brain. The objective is to have the therapist and client work together to connect inner visceral sensations to emotions and help them explore these emotions/feelings in a curious manner, actively combatting the individual's natural propensity to avoid or be numb to trauma-related emotions and feelings. This can assist in reinhabiting the body, which is the essence of feeling alive.

Examples of activities that help to understand inner visceral sensations:

1. Use a body map.
2. Use the vocabulary of sensation word list to help identify the sensations felt in the body.
3. Try to match the bodily sensation to the raw emotion systems using the table below and identify how they may be connected to emerging higher-order emotions.

Linking Sensations to Feelings and Emotions

Bodily sensations associated with emotional systems (Note: This will be different for each client, and you can have them fill this out.)	Raw emotional systems (defined by Panksepp, 1998)	Complex emerging emotions (reflective brain)
	SEEKING/ expectancy system	Interest, frustration, craving, longing
	RAGE/anger	Anger, irritability, hatred
	FEAR/anxiety	Anxiety, worry
	LUST/sexuality	Eroticism, jealousy
	CARE/nurturance	Nurturance, love, attraction
	PANIC	Separation distress, sadness, guilt/shame
	PLAY/joy	Joy, glee, happy

Vocabulary of Sensation (Ogden & Fisher, 2015)

achy	congested	flaccid	jumbly	radiating	trembling
airy	constricted	floaty	knotted	sharp	twitchy
bloated	cold	fluid	light	shivery	vibrating
blocked	cool	flushed	moist	shuddering	warm
breathless	damp	fluttery	nauseous	sore	weak
bubbly	dense	fuzzy	numb	stiff	wobbly
burning	dizzy	goosebumps	paralyzed	suffocating	
buzzy	dull	heavy	pins/needles	sweaty	
chills	electric	hollow	prickly	tense	
churning	empty	hot	puffy	thick	
clammy	energized	itchy	quaking	ticklish	
clenched	faint	jerky	quivery	tight	

7

Feeling the World
through the Senses
THE SHATTERED UNIVERSE AFTER TRAUMA

Seeing is believing . . . but feeling is truth
—THOMAS FULLER (1732)

Salience in a World Full of Noise:
Attending to What's Important

Although past research has placed an emphasis on understanding isolated sensory experiences, no sensory event is unisensory. A primary role of the nervous system is to fuse together information from multiple senses, thus enabling us to experience the full palette of sensations. For example, imagine eating crème brûlée. Your taste buds salivate when smelling its signature aroma of vanilla and carmelized sugar. Simultaneously, you hear the crust crack when tapped with a spoon and see the gentle movement of the smooth cream following the break. Although all of these senses are stimulated while eating this dessert, they are each just a part of the scene's larger tapestry that includes the chatter of restaurant patrons, the pattern of the tablecloth, the air's inherent scent, and the feeling of your clothes against your skin. However, these background sensations are irrelevant to your experience of this decadent dessert, and you easily ignore the waiter passing by your table as you take your first bite.

Noise, a cluster of irrelevant sensory signals, is present at every moment of our lives, and our body, mind, and brain have evolved to sift through these sensations and extract the most salient aspects to meet our current situational demands. In stark contrast, traumatic experiences can significantly limit our capacity to discern salient information from noise. Traumatized individuals lose the ability to

107

distinguish the sensory experience of eating crème brûlée from background noise, leaving them in a persistent state of hypervigilance. They become conditioned to scan every sensory detail in the environment, a hallmark of altered salience detection in the aftermath of trauma.

The Cocktail Party Effect: Top-Down and Bottom-Up Attentional Processes Influence What Is Salient to Us

Have you ever tried to engage in a conversation with a person at a noisy event? Our attention to a chosen auditory stimulus throughout a background cacophony of noises is known as the cocktail party effect (Handel, 1993). This metaphor suggests that we filter out background noise to focus on not only the most pertinent but also the physically closest auditory information. To focus on the critical parts of a conversation at a cocktail party, you need to consciously engage your attention to follow the flow of the conversation and make meaning of its most important elements. However, if a glass breaks in the background, this sudden noise overrides the conversation at hand and reorients our attention to the potential danger. This example illustrates the bidirectional stream through which we attend to salient stimuli in our brain. Here, consciously attending to the conversation would be an example of engaging top-down voluntary attention mechanisms mediated by the reflective brain. However, the sudden noise from the glass breaking represents a potential threat that enters at the level of the survival brain to generate a quick involuntary orienting reaction through bottom-up processing. If you remember Jeremy in Chapter 2, attending a cocktail party would be an intolerable experience. His capacity to filter out background noise from salient information is severely compromised due to his intense hypervigilance, where he feels that everything in the environment needs to be closely monitored at all times. The intensity of the collective noise compounded by anticipation of threat is too overwhelming and consequently often avoided by Jeremy.

Multisensory Integration: How Your External and Internal Senses Generate a Unified Picture of the World

When analyzing the external environment, the scene's exteroceptive sensory components are perceived at different speeds. For example, light travels at approximately 300 million meters per second while sound travels at only about 340 meters per second (Bell, 1880). However, if you are speaking with someone close by, you will likely not notice the different speeds of light and sound. This is due to the fact that our brain, mind, and body are highly adept in binding sensory information together in time and space. The process of encoding, transforming, and interpreting information into a single unified experience is one of the brain's most important functions (Stein & Stanford, 2008). We describe below the process of how our brain makes sense of the world around us.

Have you ever wondered how your senses, which speak different languages (e.g., sight, touch, auditory, gustatory, scent), create a unified experience of the world? First, all sensory stimuli in our environment predominantly travel to the survival layer of the brain (with the exception of smell). This is where the sensory input exists in its purest form and begins to fuse together with other incoming sensations. As this information travels through the brain, there is further extraction of salient sensory information and filtering of what is irrelevant so as to conserve the energy needed for more intricate functions that optimize human potential. These higher-order, energy-consuming processes include building social bonds, negotiating an ever-changing environment, and planning and organizing for our future. This intricate extraction process is how we derive the pleasures, and agonies, of our existence.

The vestibular system provides a landscape for the other sensory systems to be mapped onto and acts as a binding agent to create a unified sensory experience in space and time. Vestibular feedback then modulates the weighting of other types of exteroceptive sensory information, particularly given its role in maintaining our equilibrium in the face of a constant inflow of sensory stimuli. Here, external signals are always processed against the backdrop of our internal model of gravity and interoceptive sensory information, informing us of our bodily state and thus coloring how we perceive information from the outside world.

As each type of exteroceptive sensory stimulus enters the brain, it is weighted differently depending on its strength and survival relevance in relation to the other senses. The weighting of the senses has a direct effect on how they are bound together to form how we perceive the world through multisensory integration. For example, if the intensity of each exteroceptive sense is faint, it is easier to facilitate multisensory integration where the sum of the multiple senses forms a cohesive perspective more powerful than its individual sensory components (for a visual description, see Figure 7.1). By contrast, when a unisensory modality is weighted as stronger in relation to the other senses, multisensory integration is compromised because sensory processing is biased toward the strongest and most salient sense.

In dangerous situations, we may weigh unisensory input more strongly to enhance our chances of survival. For instance, our sense of hearing is heightened when we are in a dark alleyway, and visual feedback about our position in space becomes paramount when we are losing our balance. This phenomenon is observed in Jeremy when the sound of the fireworks extinguishes the strength of all other sensory stimuli. His attention becomes directed solely toward the sound of the fireworks at the expense of experiencing the full palette of sensations that accompany fireworks (e.g., colors, design, smell) or attuning to intimate moments with his children. The sound of the fireworks overrides any other sensory stimuli

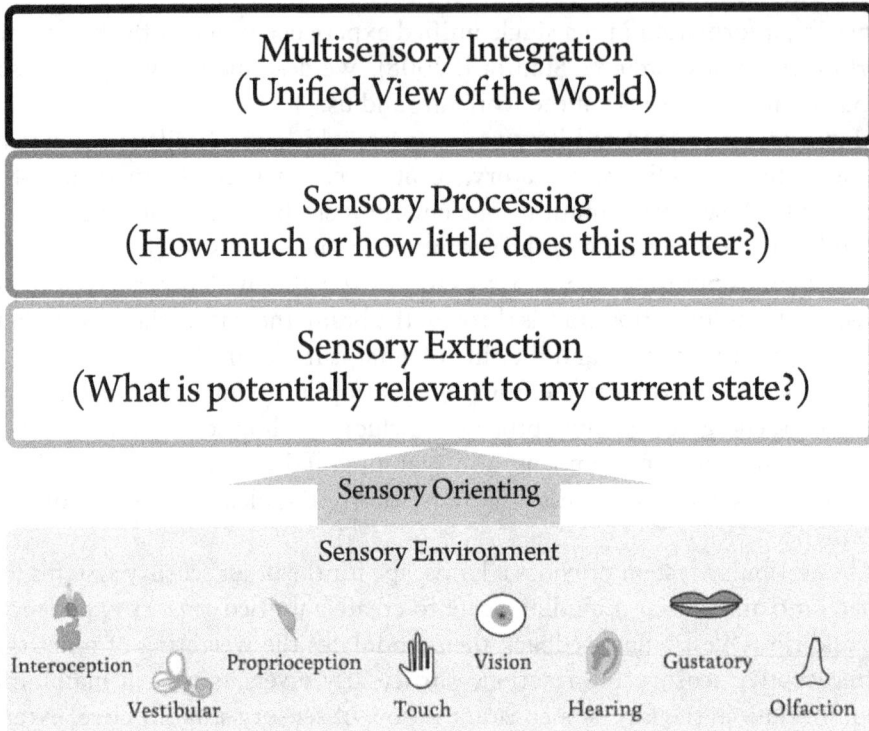

FIGURE 7.1. How the brain anticipates and integrates incoming sensory information.

at that moment and could precipitate a flashback, where Jeremy loses his sense of time and space in the present while reliving the rocket attack in the form of vivid visual and auditory sensory flashes. This multisensory integrative breakdown corresponded with a disruption to his sensory equilibrium, causing him to lose the bearings that anchor his body in time and space. Ultimately, Jeremy's children were left feeling frightened from their overwhelmed and disconnected parent.

"When I Feel Off Balance, I Don't Feel Safe in the World": Hyper- and Hyposensitivity Because the World Is Unstable

At any moment, an underlying, ineffable understanding of how to move our bodies to effectively navigate the external environment is paramount for experiencing the full palette of sensations. This understanding is facilitated by efficient vestibular and somatosensory integration at the level of the survival brain, which serves to modulate or balance signals coming from the external world in light of this contextualized bodily information. When we feel that the signals informing us of where our body is in space, how to move our body, and how to keep our own body safe are untrustworthy, our literal and figurative senses of balance are off-kilter. As a result, we may rely more on exteroceptive sensations (vision, touch, hearing) to navigate the external world. This imbalance can result in chronic states of physical and emotional instability. Without a solid anchor to the body and reliable access to its capacities, the ability to integrate external sensory information into the body schema and sense of bodily self in the present moment suffers.

Individual differences in hyper- and hyposensitivity to external sensory input after trauma must be considered:

- *Hypersensitivity to exteroceptive sensations.* If our body registers that threat may be imminent from the external world, our nervous system can shift to lower our thresholds for external sensory input, thus heightening exteroceptive sensory sensitivities. From our previous case example in Chapter 4, Lola was on high alert for external threats due to her history of abuse as a young child, corresponding to her high reactivity to sounds, lights, smells, and touch. In other words, her heightened vigilance for external sensory input related to potential threats precluded multisensory integration, disturbed her sensory equilibrium, and prevented her from ever experiencing a calm and easeful internal state. Furthermore, without solid integration of body-based sensations during early development with a secure attachment figure, such as being held and rocked with care when distressed, Lola experienced a greater need to rely on exteroceptive sensations to navigate her external world. These exteroceptive hypersensitivities are adaptive yet overwhelming and come at the expense of Lola safely inhabiting her physical body.

- *Depersonalization.* Alternatively, for some who experienced inescapable threat from the outside, such as rape, trauma-relevant external stimuli, such as touch or the smell of a perpetrator's cologne, may prompt detachment from the potentially lethal external sensory world, resulting in depersonalization.

- *Hyperfixation on internal bodily cues.* In another instance, a hyperfixation on internal bodily cues may ensue if threats are unexpectedly generated from our internal world, such as overwhelming visceral anguish from confusing or disorienting emotional events. This is an example of lowered thresholds for bodily signals, such as visceral information and pain. This hyperfixation on the internal body can hinder the processing of exteroceptive information, contributing to derealization symptoms.

Hence, different multisensory processing imbalances may emerge depending upon each individual's coping patterns. For some, fluctuations between hyper- and hyposensitivity may also occur. These individual differences in arousal and behavioral responses to exteroceptive and interoceptive sensory information make it difficult for researchers and clinicians to draw meaningful conclusions for any one diagnosis—thus, an individualized approach to treatment is critical.

Exteroception after Trauma:
The Interior World Mirrors the External World

The way in which we perceive sensations from the external world is dependent upon the inner state of our bodies. Imagine a time when you felt calm and at peace with yourself. As you walk to work, a car drives by through a large puddle and splashes you. You are slightly startled but quickly recover and even laugh with your coworkers as you explain why your coat is wet when you arrive. Such an inner state allowed you to take the unexpected wetness with stride and to feel patient with the driver of the car. Then, imagine an inner world where sensations and feelings of being overwhelmed, threatened, and eaten up inside predominate. In the same scenario with the car, you are extremely perturbed by the sudden splash and yell obscenities at the driver. You feel so overstimulated that you must turn around and go home to change.

Such an agonizing and tortuous inner state led to the experience of the world as unsafe and where people cannot be trusted, thus leaving the individual feeling deserted and slighted. Unfortunately, this reflects the reality of many traumatized individuals that feeling safe both within oneself and with one's surroundings becomes a foreign concept. Importantly, this can lead to a loss of attunement with one's surroundings and feelings that nothing and no one can be trusted. This brings us back to Chapter 6, where we discussed that in order to minimize unpredictability, the traumatized individual consistently expects danger to occur. Consequently, they lose the capacity to adapt flexibly to nonthreatening situations because the body has adjusted to a new persistent steady state of threat. Here, hypervigilance and paranoia often dominate the traumatized individual's life, and the world is perceived as a perpetually dangerous place.

Derealization:
When the World Becomes Insurmountable

When we perceive our reality as an insurmountable threat, psychological escape becomes the only option. This perception can precipitate a profoundly protective disconnect not only from one's own body but also from the threatening surroundings. *If it's not real, it's not happening.* In cases of severe developmental trauma, this can involve a complete blocking of all sensory information arising from within the body to the point where the individual can only feel the existence of their body through forceful sensory input, including self-injury, such as cutting or burning oneself. Individuals can lose the capacity to feel some of the most life-sustaining sensations, including hunger, thirst, and pain. This loss of access to inner sensations and feelings has a powerful effect on how the world is perceived. It may seem distorted or utterly dampened in its sensory content to the point where things seem unreal. The individual may not even be able to perceive other people as real or present. This often leaves the traumatized individual feeling robbed of a sense of belonging, as they are unable to access "the other" through nurturing and healing social connection. However, when the absence of "the other" is a reality, such as in cases of severe childhood neglect, this can be a lifesaving accommodation made by the mind, brain, and body; lacking full perception of the damaging "other" softens the blow of their absence.

The following quote by a severely neglected developmental trauma survivor eloquently illustrates the experience of a profoundly altered interplay between intero- and exteroception.

"Interoception is to me the felt experience of living in a body, no, in my body. I experienced my body only in its deficits or its injuries. I couldn't jump rope. I fell down some concrete stairs and was knocked out. I burned my arm. These were the primary sources of information I had that there was a body. There was no end to my nervous system; my nerve endings never ended. My therapy for many years could be understood as my attempt to recruit another, to get the therapist to show up in ways that I could hear and feel in my body. The existence of me in my body depended entirely on my establishing his existence. These were contingent and probably nearly co-arising realities, but my felt sense is that there was a sequence: First came the parent, then came the child. For me to exist I needed to know that he existed, and to know it again and again. I had to come up against him and he had to meet that endlessly. He would disappear almost as soon as I left his office. I believed that I dropped out of his mind and then again I had only my overwhelming feeling states to suggest my existence. *They were unboundaried and, in that, unbearable.* Every session was the origin story. If he didn't exist, I didn't exist, so I had to make sure he showed up, that I could feel him. I felt like a blind kitten. I sought him out in the dark. I couldn't understand his words. I needed the reality of his body. . . . This depth of encounter gave me my body and with it a sense of self: self and other, self from other, self in other. It provided skin. And he was at first the focal point of exteroception. I had to experience that there was an inner and then an outer and then to feel where they met to make me and my experience approximate real."

This individual's experience highlights how exteroceptive stimuli explored through therapeutic sensory-based interactions (e.g., soothing voice) help the individual develop interoception, where they perceive themselves existing in the eyes of another for the first time. Once this relationship is established and the dynamic between interoception and exteroception is felt, the therapist can then mirror the client, co-regulate, and hold the client's intense positive and negative affective states.

Re-Creating Safety in the Outside World
Using a Therapeutic Setting

Importance of Co-Regulation in Trauma-Focused Interventions

Co-regulation refers to the way in which the nervous system of one individual regulates the nervous system of another, making it an interpersonal process that allows for attunement between two individuals (Bornstein & Esposito, 2023; Butler & Randall, 2013). Specifically, it helps foster a deep connection of felt safety via subconscious interactions between the two nervous systems. Co-regulation allows the infant to experience the felt sense of being soothed as the caregiver tolerates and holds their distress while remaining regulated in their own nervous system. Through this process, a regulated adult acts as a solid foundation to ease the distress of the child, forming a dyadic bidirectional emotional system that oscillates between high and low arousal states to maintain an optimal emotional state (Ferrer & Helm, 2013; Fosha, 2001). Co-regulation is a prerequisite for self-regulation, which is one of the most important developmental outcomes of a secure upbringing. The principles of self-regulation of affective states are therefore "taught" within the scaffolding of another (Siegel, 2009). For those who lacked a reliable caregiver in childhood to form this dyadic system, the therapeutic environment and relationship can use co-regulation as a means to teach self-regulation.

Co-regulation in childhood inherently utilizes exteroceptive sensory information, including auditory pitch (e.g., singing a lullaby), touch or swaddling, rhythmic movements (bouncing a baby), and shared visual stimuli. In a therapeutic setting, the therapist may offer opportunities for similar kinds of soothing sensory input, such as a Lycra swing that allows for rhythmic movements and the sense of being held, to support co-regulation and ultimately foster the development of self-regulation capacities (Warner et al., 2020).

The therapist may mimic a client's engagement with an external sensory-rich object as a means to match their internal affective state, attuning to the client's nervous system and implicitly guiding the client toward self-regulation (see Bridging to Practice 7 for additional guidance about how to implement these strategies in a therapeutic setting). For example, a client may be sitting in a rocking chair or bouncing on an exercise ball, engaging in a rhythmic movement at their own pace. Here, the therapist could engage in the same movement and mirror their pace while remaining attuned to the client's arousal and emotional states. This synchrony between the client and therapist can engender a sense of feeling seen, which may be a new experience for traumatized individuals who often feel alone and misunderstood. *When we are seen, we are not alone.*

Healing from the Inside Out: Toward Feeling Safe and Sound

Safe and Sound Protocol (SSP) core, an algorithm-driven filtered music program developed by Stephen W. Porges, is a noninvasive bottom-up therapy that also uses rhythmic movement to train the nervous system to be receptive to cues of safety and to downregulate innate defensive actions. As the client listens to the various frequencies of the SSP, the protocol has been proposed to target the dynamic between the facial nerve and the vagus nerve, two cranial nerves that branch off from the survival brain. In the context of this book, we hypothesize an expansive neural mechanism beyond the vagus and facial nerves that fits with the context of sensory processing more broadly, including critical structures in the survival brain where sensation, raw emotion, and arousal meet. These include the reticular activating system, the inferior colliculus, the superior colliculus, and the periaqueductal gray.

The SSP is likely to also stimulate the auditory and vestibular systems using focused pitch frequencies that emulate the prosody of human speech and social connection, which can be both stress inducing and soothing. For example, its frequency can be emotionally and autonomically dysregulating if a traumatized individual had limited access to a soothing voice while growing up, or if they received conflicted signals from a sometimes nurturing, sometimes abusive caregiver. The SSP uses musical rhythms to help establish the body's inner metronome, providing an inner rhythm that can regulate fluctuating arousal and emotional states. As the patient listens to the various frequencies, we hypothesize that the sensory input from the SSP reaches the inferior and superior colliculi, as well as the periaqueductal gray in the survival brain. This input travels through the reticular formation, a key region where arousal meets raw affect and sensation. From here, it is relayed throughout mind and body as integrated sensory-affective information. The SSP protocol aids with autonomic regulation to help downregulate defensiveness and attenuate negative raw affect experienced at the level of periaqueductal gray and the reticular formation. Here, the reticular formation is a key intersection between brain and body, as it is integral for translating sensory information to the emotional learning and reflective brain layers, as well as influencing visceral and musculoskeletal processes through the vagus nerve and reticulospinal somatosensory tracts. Vibrations from sound frequencies also stimulate the vestibular system, which plays a critical role in balancing our inner and outer worlds.

CASE EXAMPLE: The Safe and Sound Protocol

BY LIZ CHARLES, MD

In 2018, Liz Charles delivered the SSP in person to her client, Martha. Martha is a mother of three in her late 50s with a history of complex trauma, which includes emotional and sexual abuse from three generations of her family, as well as ritual abuse and domestic violence from her ex-husband. She suffered from prolonged ill health and chronic fatigue for many years as an adult, and she searched desperately for some respite, unaware of her trauma and its impact. She finally accessed

kind and skilled support from both a somatic therapist and a person-centered psychotherapist, and her brain and body slowly released the locked-in memories and
emotions. She gradually processed the disturbing hidden memories held in her
body, which Martha remembers as a "deeply disturbed time with relentless twists
and turns." Martha started to experience significant benefits both physically and
mentally but still longed for greater relief and decided to try SSP.

Aware of Martha's history, vulnerability, and tendency to be overwhelmed
by anything new, Liz worked closely with Martha to prepare for the SSP listening sessions. Time was given for Martha to settle into each session before careful
titration of SSP. Martha also maintained regular contact with her therapist for
ongoing support.

During the third session of SSP, Liz noticed Martha suddenly lost attention
and energy, so she stopped the music. Martha seemed disoriented and shaken but
said she was fine. Recognizing that Martha had entered a deep shutdown state
and dissociated, Liz spoke quietly to reassure her and gradually Martha became
more present again. Martha described the experience:

> "It was weird. I was in my familiar place of deepest darkest haunted nothing-
> ness, where I'd always felt totally isolated and alone. But this time, it felt so
> different; there was a gentle caring presence of someone with me, next to me;
> it felt so special, warm, and lovely."

The next day a momentous event then happened to Martha: "I was at home
doing nothing in particular when I suddenly landed in my body. It was crazy.
Everything was different, I was no longer floating above and watching myself.
Is this how everyone else lives? This is easy!" Martha still clearly remembers
this exact moment in time and space, "It was so real, a one-way journey into my
body—a life-changing moment."

This opened a whole new world for Martha. "It might sound weird but before
this I knew I had a body because I could see it, but now I actually feel connected
to my body and part of it!" As Liz and Martha continued slow titration of SSP,
Liz guided Martha in building a regular self-care routine of sensory and breathing activities to support and strengthen her nervous system. Martha was surprised
to find she enjoyed these: "I can now see that my body can be helpful and give
me strength. This is so different to before when I would get so frustrated that my
body kept letting me down."

Four years later, Martha reported an extraordinary experience:

> "I was on vacation with a close friend, relaxing and rocking on a porch swing,
> when suddenly all my senses became intense. It was like a dark veil lifted
> and I was seeing the world in technicolor. Colors were more vivid, sounds
> became crystal clear, and my skin became sensitive to touch in a way I'd
> never experienced before. My whole body felt different. I felt new sensations

in my toes, which then moved up through my feet and into my body. It was amazingly wonderful. I felt so much more connected to my body, connected to the ground. I could feel energy flowing through me, and my whole body felt more alive. I wanted to stretch, and I felt like I was moving with so much more freedom and feeling of space, especially in my hips and pelvis. It felt like a whole new awakening.

"I then had a meltdown, with an intense body reaction that vividly reminded me of a terrible time when my father inflicted the most horrendous abuse on me when I was 3. I sobbed and sobbed and held onto my friend. It was so good to have her hugs and support. After that, it all felt so different. It was amazing. It felt like real inside-out healing. I was no longer scared to be in my body. I felt like a new me."

Martha's attitude toward herself then changed fundamentally:

"I can now treat myself with kindness and compassion. I can now appreciate all that my body and mind suffered and endured, and I'm no longer ashamed. I can barely believe I survived so much. It's really different to be so aware of sensations in my body now, and great to be in touch with my gut feeling. It's such a relief to have times now when I can let go and relax and connect with a deep part of myself—a peaceful joy I had always longed for."

Martha further notes:

"But on the flip side, the increased sensations in my body can sometimes feel overwhelming. Sometimes I miss the foggy numbness. I struggle to deal with intense feelings of anxiety in my body and it's really tempting to avoid situations that cause them. I have to work hard to remind myself there is not some impending doom and disaster lurking around the corner."

This case exemplifies the therapist's commitment to ensure SSP is titrated with each client to maximize the effectiveness of this potent tool using her "Sensitive Approach: Client at the Core" method for clients with trauma histories and chronic illnesses. A trusting relationship is built with each client and psychoeducation is offered to encourage understanding of their physiological state and associated features. Various supportive activities are used during pauses in listening sessions to allow any shifts to emerge, evolve, and integrate, and clients are encouraged to use these activities as ongoing resources to strengthen their nervous systems in their day-to-day lives.

Martha says:

"I feel like a different person—so much younger with far more energy. I feel connected to my inner and outer worlds in ways I couldn't have begun to imagine. I'm still getting used to this new world of it being okay to feel, and to know my world isn't going to collapse around me. I still have the memories, but I'm no longer confused, and they don't destroy me like they used to. It's wonderful to have this sense of inner peace now, and to even have moments of hope and confidence for my future."

Going Outward to Go Inward: Expanding the Dynamic Between Exteroception and Interoception for Trauma Processing

Eye Movement Desensitization and Reprocessing

EMDR is an intervention that uses eye movements or other forms of bilateral stimulation to help individuals alleviate distress and dampen negative affect while reprocessing traumatic memories (Shapiro & Maxfield, 2002). Here, the client is asked to focus on a traumatic memory while simultaneously experiencing bilateral stimulation, which is thought to desensitize the affective sensations associated with these memories and subsequently alter the way they are processed and stored. As described above, voluntary eye movements are mediated by the dorsal attention network in the reflective brain, where activation of the frontal eye fields leads to concurrent activation of brain regions responsible for emotion regulation (Harricharan et al., 2019). With use of bilateral stimulation within a safe therapeutic setting, the individual is desensitized to the intense affect over multiple sessions and interoceptive and exteroceptive sensations associated with the traumatic memory. Reducing the emotional intensity of the traumatic memory can allow for its reprocessing and help shape it into a historical event, one that is part of one's personal life journey rather than an overwhelming terror in the present.

Deep Brain Reorienting

DBR is a novel psychotherapeutic approach that harnesses our burgeoning understanding of the survival brain's neurophysiological responses to traumatic events (Corrigan & Christie-Sands, 2020). Given that the survival brain operates quickly and beneath our conscious awareness to conserve energy and preserve our safety, targeting these survival responses may be key in getting to the root of trauma. In particular, the survival brain is positioned to act as a relay center between the brain and the body, suggesting that targeting this region through DBR may act directly on internal bodily events (and our experience of them).

Upon retrieving a traumatic memory or reminder in a therapeutic setting, the DBR clinician guides the individual in focusing on an orienting tension that naturally arises in the head and neck. This orienting tension is thought to be elicited by the superior colliculus of the survival brain in preparation to turn the eyes and head toward or away from a threat (Corneil, Munoz, Chapman, Admans, & Cushing, 2008; Corneil, Olivier, & Munoz, 2002). This orienting tension is noticed and deepened with guidance from a trained therapist and acts as a grounding anchor for the rest of the therapeutic process. Once this anchor is solidified, signals from the superior colliculus may activate the locus coeruleus, also in the survival brain, to elicit an emotional "shock" response. This shock response may manifest somatically as trembling or shaking, a pulling sensation behind the eyes, or a bracing tension in the upper muscles of the back. DBR is the only current psychotherapeutic approach to address this shock response, which needs to be fully expressed and processed in the context of the therapeutic relationship to arrive at the raw, visceral sensations at the level of the periaqueductal gray (FEAR, RAGE, GRIEF, etc.) in a regulated manner. These raw visceral sensations, interoceptive in nature, may then be noticed and processed with clarity while grounded in the physical body through the orienting tension. Eight sessions of DBR have been shown to significantly decrease PTSD-related symptom severity (Kearney, Corrigan, et al., 2023), suggesting that reorienting the physical body to the present through mindful attention to relevant internally generated sensations may attenuate and render tolerable the visceral affective responses that plague traumatized individuals.

A DBR participant, initially skeptical about a treatment approach so different from what she was used to in talk therapy, reported the following:

"Like anyone else, I had my skepticism and my preconceptions about how the session would go. After all, I never considered myself to have that severe of trauma. Sure, my parents lost their tempers. Any parent gets frustrated with their kid when they talk back and don't listen. I brought up a particularly clear memory of my father coming toward me with both arms outstretched, his hands rigidly shaped to perfectly encapsulate my soft, vulnerable neck. The memory of that moment laid crisp in my mind, although what happened after goes blank. I decided to use this moment, since I had recently had a strong reaction when my partner touched my neck—I became extremely defensive and angry. Logically, or so I thought, I predicted that DBR would bring up tension in my neck. I was wrong. Tension crept into the muscles around my eyes. My attempts to rationalize everything kept creeping back in. 'It must be because I had winced,' I thought.

"My therapist gently reminded me to return to my body, to keep holding on to the facial tension. Eventually I felt a seemingly separate tightness emerge across my upper back, as if to brace for some sort of impact. It was unexpected. But it started to make sense. Suddenly, a tickling, nervous feeling crept into my abdomen. My therapist guided me back to the tension around my eyes, then my back. 'Stay with it.' It felt uncomfortable, but important. It had things to say. I kept my eyes closed and listened. Eventually she guided the nervous gut feeling into the sequence. 'What are you feeling?,' she asked. 'I feel like I want to get up and move. I want to get up and run.'

"After what felt like a few minutes, the therapist gently told me it had been an hour and that the session was concluding. She asked if I had any new insights, new perspectives. I said, 'I always want to go for a run when I'm stressed. Actually, I would run every day of my life if I could to keep my stress levels down. I run on injuries, I run in the frigid winter, I run at 4:00 A.M. before an early flight instead of getting much-needed sleep.' Was this 'compulsive exercising' a disorder of my brain, or was it a compulsion to act on the uncomfortable feelings that arise whenever this sequence is triggered, anytime I feel like I'm losing control? I hadn't started out focusing on my exercise addiction, but it emerged from somewhere deep within. I learned more in that hour of silence than I had learned in 16 years of talking about it."

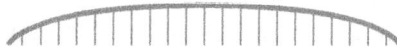

BRIDGING TO PRACTICE 7

Sensory Hygiene:
Where the Window of Tolerance Meets Sensory Mindfulness

Sensory mindfulness refers to the capacity to be consciously aware of the sensations encountered in our external and internal worlds on a moment-to-moment basis. Conscious awareness is not necessarily focused attention—rather, it requires a level of reflection on how all types of external sensations interact with one's internal state of the body. One's degree of sensory mindfulness directly impacts how they navigate their surroundings, where many traumatized individuals can embody a robotic autopilot state that is detached and alienated from their closest social bonds and nature itself.

The goal is to reconnect and fortify the traumatized individual's inner sensations with external sensations experienced in the outer world at a tolerable pace. For example, having an individual notice small movements while seated on a physio ball or sensations in their muscles when they pick up a weighted object may bring conscious awareness to safe sensations in the present. This can help counterbalance the persistent anticipation of threat based on terrors from the past. Embracing these safe sensations in a therapeutic setting can help individuals track how they move throughout the window of tolerance during the session (Siegel, 1999; for a discussion of the window of tolerance, see Chapter 4 and Plate 4.2). Outside of the session, clients can use Figure 7.2 to monitor their arousal levels throughout the day and begin to enhance their awareness of how sensory experiences interact with their arousal level.

To maximize therapeutic gain, it is ideal for the client to reach the fluid zones of the window of tolerance because they can notice more subtle signs in their shifts in arousal rather than feeling fully immersed in a dysregulated state. It is important for the therapist and client to *both* be aware and able to identify when the

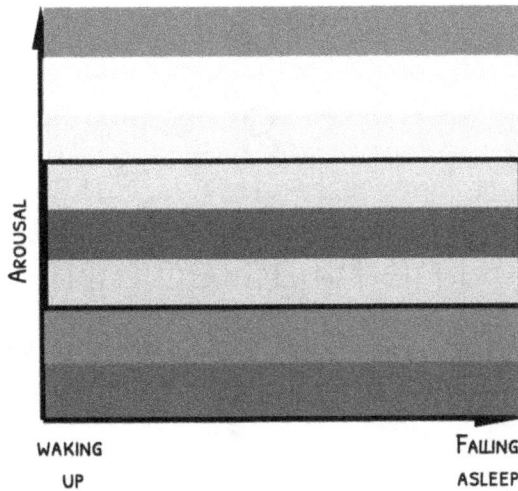

FIGURE 7.2. Map for monitoring arousal levels throughout the day.

client enters the fluid zone, which is a highly individualized process. Here are some signs that may be indicative of a client entering a fluid zone of arousal:

1. A feeling of discomfort arising while an individual remains grounded in the present. As an example, this may be a feeling of slight tension without feeling overwhelmed.

2. For the therapist, this may feel like a strenuous task because it requires additional co-regulation to prevent the client from overshooting the fluid zone and entering a state of hyper-/hypoarousal.

3. The therapist may feel an urge to ground the client by repeating "You are safe, you are in the present, and/or nobody is going to hurt you." However, this needs to be balanced by allowing the client to process the information internally. Here, silence can be your friend as long as you can be sure the client is firmly grounded in the present.

4. The goal of the therapist is to help keep the client attuned to their inner body while firmly grounded in the present for as long as they can tolerate it. Initially, this may last for as little as a couple of seconds. Remember, a slower pace can often get you there faster.

8

The Hijacked Self

OVERCOMING THE COMPULSION
TO REPEAT THE TRAUMA

The greatest hazard of all, losing one's self, can occur very quietly
in the world, as if it were nothing at all. No other loss can occur
so quietly; any other loss—an arm, a leg, five dollars, a wife,
etc.—is sure to be noticed.
—SØREN KIERKEGAARD (1849/1980)

Many traumatized individuals have a seemingly unshakable feeling that they are "damaged," "defective," or "broken." Alterations to the survival brain's functioning in the wake of trauma disrupts an individual's capacity to effectively and efficiently process proprioceptive, somatosensory, vestibular, and interoceptive information, which inform us of our body's current state and capacities. Though speculative, this disruption may be due to their prior experiences with helplessness during an overwhelming, traumatic event. Repeated instances of traumatic experiences, such as in the case of chronic childhood traumatization, may further solidify this inexplicable feeling of defectiveness emanating in part from survival brain-level disruptions (Nakazawa, 2015; Teicher et al., 2016). This may explain why so many traumatized individuals state that they can tell themselves "consciously" that they are good and worthy, but they cannot seem to escape the deep feelings of worthlessness, helplessness, shame, and guilt that arise any time they experience a reminder or theme from the past (Platt & Freyd, 2015).

Connecting the Dots for the Full Picture:
An Introduction to Brain Networks

Your brain accounts for about 20% of your energy demands despite its small size relative to the body (2%), necessitating structures and networks that can be as efficient as possible while enhancing function (Raichle & Gusnard, 2002). The adaptive process of plasticity, described in Hebb's (2002) saying "what fires together, wires together," summarizes the incredible process by which our brain dynamically adapts to become more efficient in the face of new information, including input from senseless, agonizing, and life-threatening experiences. If we were to juxtapose the physical brains of a nontraumatized and a traumatized person, we would not be able to distinguish the two by the naked eye. The brain is not broken; it has undergone "functional" adaptations to persevere despite unspeakably cruel or devastating circumstances.

One way to measure communication patterns in the brain is through functional connectivity, which is based on blood flow to its different regions over a certain period of time. During these timeframes, computational measures decipher which brain regions show synchronous activity, or similar patterns of blood flow in response to certain tasks. Therefore, functional connectivity is a measure of connection strength among different brain regions and reflects patterns of how brain regions fire together (Shine et al., 2019). The latter represents the foundation of what is referred to as a network. All critical functions in the brain are represented by networks, including attention, planning, memory, movement, social connection, and introspection.

There are several foundational networks in the brain that underlie these crucial functions, including:

- The central executive network (e.g., cognitive tasks, planning)
- The salience network (e.g., attending to the environment, coordinating movements)
- The default mode network (DMN; e.g., introspection, sense of self, memory, social connection; Menon, 2011; Seeley et al., 2007)
- The sensorimotor network (e.g., conscious somatosensory perception; voluntary movement, movement planning)

When we perform certain actions, it would not be energy efficient for all brain networks to be online. For example, reading this book predominantly requires your central executive network. Therefore, certain brain regions are more connected, or fire more synchronously, during certain tasks. In this chapter, we focus on how the DMN and the sensorimotor network are disrupted after trauma. As you will read, the brains of trauma survivors show exceptional adaptations to functional networks as a way to respond and adapt to life's catastrophes, which is a testament to the immense resiliency of the human mind, brain, body, and spirit. Despite coming from different walks of life, the brain networks of trauma survivors often resemble one another, demonstrating common survival-oriented transformations. The brain's innate capacity to adjust to deal with adversity also means that it can adapt to embrace safety and stability; it is not solely wired to survive but also to thrive and reach inner peace through neuroplasticity.

The Brain Identity of the Self in the Aftermath of Trauma

The experience of psychological trauma can have a profound impact on our identity and our sense of self (Fisher, 2017; Fosha, 2013; Frewen et al., 2020; Lanius et al., 2020). Chronic developmental trauma often prevents individuals from ever forming a coherent sense of who they are in the world, a critical ingredient in the agentive pursuit of our hopes and dreams. Without a solid sense of self, the ability to project this self into the future is impossible. The void left where the sense of self could have existed can be unbearable. The feeling that the self does not exist is very much related to the subjective somatic experience of being unable to feel one's bodily edges and thus not knowing where one begins and where one ends. These somatic boundaries are necessary elements for a coherent sense of self and a knowing that one exists in the world. Where does this ability to "feel our edges" originate? One can argue that the early attachment relationship plays a fundamental role in forming the very essence of the felt experience of who we are (Schore, 2003; Siegel, 2020). Here, the caregiver both physically and mentally holds the infant, where the mind and body of the infant are held closely by the mind and body of the caregiver. The securely attached infant has their needs attended to and their emotional states mirrored. This overt caregiver reflection forms the base for self-reflection later in development. Through the tender touch and movement shared between child and caregiver, the foundations of felt bodily existence begin to form. If these basic human needs remain unmet, as is the case in chronic neglect and/or abuse, the individual is left with a profound deficit in the foundational requirements for the development of a coherent sense of self. An unbearable emptiness comes to exist where the self could have been.

In the case of adult-onset trauma where the individual had the chance to develop a more or less coherent sense of self, they are often left feeling as though "I am not me anymore," "I have lost my sense of self and my identity," and "I will never be able to feel normal emotions again." Somatic accounts representative of a felt bodily experience of a loss of self can include "I feel dead inside," "I am always on edge," and "I feel detached from my body" (Cox, Fesik, Kimmelman, Luo, & Der, 2014; Fisher, 2017; Foa, Ehlers, Clark, Tolin, & Orsillo, 1999). Moreover, traumatized individuals are regularly plagued by physical symptoms, including breathing difficulties, gastrointestinal disturbances, and chronic pain (Graham, Searle, Van Hooff, Lawrence-Wood, & McFarlane, 2019), which can impact significantly how these persons experience who they are and what they are capable of.

The sense of self has been suggested to be neurobiologically represented by the DMN, a group of brain regions nestled along the midline of the reflective brain that actively communicate with one another during rest and introspection (Lanius et al., 2020; Menon, 2011). As a whole, the DMN plays a critical role in self-awareness, memory, future-oriented thought, embodiment, and social connection (Buckner, Andrews-Hanna, & Schacter, 2008; Frewen et al., 2020; Greicius,

Krasnow, Reiss, & Menon, 2003; Menon, 2011; Qin & Northoff, 2011; Spreng, Mar, & Kim, 2009). Specifically, the DMN comprises functional connections between the posterior cingulate cortex/precuneus, the medial prefrontal cortex, and parietal regions (Menon, 2011). The posterior cingulate cortex and the precuneus are often referred to as the posterior hub of the DMN, which plays a critical role in the reexperiencing and mental imagery aspect of a memory, whereas the medial prefrontal cortex is considered the anterior hub that is crucial in providing context while reflecting on the feelings and emotions of the past. The connections between the posterior and anterior hubs of the DMN thus form the foundation for the experience of a stable sense of self across time and into the future. The sense of self is critical in guiding a person's social interactions and deepening their social bonds (Anzellotti & Caramazza, 2017). The functional connections among areas of the DMN have been shown to be malleable, changing both in the aftermath of psychological trauma and during recovery (King et al., 2016; Lanius et al., 2015; Nicholson et al., 2020). In support of this, the neurobiological basis of one's identity and one's sense of self is indeed highly shapeable and can adapt to different environmental and social contexts.

Default-Mode Network and Sensorimotor Network Disruptions in PTSD: Stuck in the Past without a Paddle

Individuals with PTSD exhibit profound disruptions in the DMN when they are asked to close their eyes and let their minds wander. This is referred to as the "resting state," a state of introspection where we are not engaged in any externally focused activity but may be thinking of past or future events. However, it has become apparent that the traumatized brain is rarely truly "at rest" but rather is in a constant state of hypervigilance, reliving, and defense. How can we make sense of the disruptions we see in the DMN or the "unrest" individuals with PTSD experience despite not actively engaging in a task? Studies examining functional connectivity within the DMN among individuals with PTSD "at rest" reveal weakened connections between the posterior and anterior hubs of the DMN, where the posterior hub remains online while the anterior hub is largely inaccessible (see Plate 8.1). The posterior DMN thus becomes the predominant hub of the network, where the mental images and emotional experiences related to past memories lack present-day contextualization via the anterior DMN (Chen & Etkin, 2013; Daniels et al., 2010; Kennis, Rademaker, van Rooij, Kahn, & Geuze, 2015; Koch, Massimini, Boly, & Tononi, 2016; Miller et al., 2017; Qin et al., 2012; Shang et al., 2014; Sripada et al., 2012). Instead, the posterior DMN is hyperconnected (overly synchronous) with the sensorimotor network, which is involved in processing somatosensory input from the physical body and eliciting motor action (Heba et al., 2017; Kearney, Terpou, et al., 2023), in individuals with PTSD during traumatic memory retrieval (see also the section "Shame and Moral Injury as Threats to the Self" later in this chapter). The traumatic memory-induced "cross-talk" between these two typically opposing functional networks, one concerned with the present and the other with the past, corresponds with increases in self-reported reliving intensity; in other words, the past seems ever present (Kearney, Terpou, et al., 2023; Plate 8.2).

Notably, studies have found that the extent of disconnection between the anterior and posterior DMN (Akiki et al., 2018; Holmes et al., 2018) and the posterior DMN and sensorimotor network coupling (Kearney, Terpou, et al., 2023) are associated with increased PTSD symptom severity. Indeed, the loss of anterior hub connections with the rest of the DMN can predispose individuals to develop PTSD (Qin et al., 2012). The loss of context provided by the anterior DMN in conjunction with heightened reliving symptoms from posterior DMN–sensorimotor network coupling destabilizes the sense of self as a continuous entity through time, compromising the capacity to voluntarily retrieve or leave the past. The traumatized individual remains stuck in a vivid past without an anchor in the present or the future.

Altered self-experience, including dissociative phenomena where individuals have a detached sense of their bodies and/or external reality, has also been associated with a reduced representation of the anterior DMN (Kearney, Terpou, et al., 2023; Tursich et al., 2015). Here, a trauma survivor describes profound alterations in such self-experience involving severe dissociative episodes:

> "The worst mirror event [experience looking in the mirror] was horrifying. I don't want that image in anyone's mind, even yours. Mostly, I was averse. I didn't 'go to' the mirror, but when I would catch a reflection, I always knew it was me. I just didn't want to see my body. I didn't feel I had a body at all. It was . . . 'an appendage.' I washed and dressed it. I had a head, but that might have been more truly felt as I had a mind. I don't think I embodied my head or face either. I rarely, if ever, used a full-length mirror. It was 'me,' but it had no meaning, and I avoided the confrontation with this confusing image and the revulsion that would follow. At some point during the first to third year of neurofeedback training, I remember I looked at my hand and realized that this was my hand. It was as I imagined; It's like an infant except that of course I knew I had these hands."

Taken together, the DMN is compartmentalized with respect to the posterior and anterior hubs of the network in individuals with PTSD, which may spur an experiential loss of self. Furthermore, the posterior hub of the DMN communicates strongly with the sensorimotor network, which maps onto more intense reliving of sensory and motor aspects of traumatic memories. Successful integration of the posterior and anterior components of the DMN, as well as uncoupling of the sensorimotor network and posterior DMN, may be crucial ingredients in the restoration and/or transformation of the self into one that can safely inhabit the body and remember, instead of relive, the past.

The Hijacked Self: The DMN under Threat in PTSD

As discussed above, the traumatized DMN exhibits drastically altered connectivity patterns both "at rest" and when retrieving a traumatic memory. These differences have been found to occur even when the trigger appears for a mere 16 milliseconds, below conscious awareness. However, a restoration of connectivity between the anterior (front) and posterior (back) hubs of the DMN is observed under conditions of threat in PTSD, thus making the traumatized DMN seem more intact. The periaqueductal gray, a brain region situated in the survival brain and critically involved in processing threat, appears to be driving this enhanced connectivity of the DMN during the subliminal exposure to trauma triggers (Terpou, Densmore, et al., 2019). The periaqueductal gray is part of the innate alarm system that specializes in coordinating fast, subconscious responses to immediate stress—instinctual responses that help you act swiftly without thinking. Here, potentially threatening sensory input from the body and the environment enters the survival brain and is quickly transmitted to the periaqueductal gray, where fast defensive responses can be initiated without the time-consuming consultation of the reflective brain (see Chapter 3). Based on animal research, this structure is heavily innervated by somatosensory input from the body and viscera and is essential in eliciting raw emotions, including fear and terror. The periaqueductal gray therefore represents a crucial subcortical hub for the subconscious processing of threat-related stimuli. The finding that the periaqueductal gray appears to reignite the DMN under threat may help to elucidate why individuals with PTSD frequently exhibit experiential links between their own traumatic experience and how they view themselves in the world. A semblance of a sense of self may *only* be garnered under threat, and the traumatic experience becomes central to their identity (for review, see Lanius et al., 2020).

Taken together, these findings help shed light on why traumatized individuals frequently seek out intensely arousing or even terrifying experiences, including sensory-seeking and reckless behavior, in order to "feel alive." For example, an interview with a person who experienced chronic developmental trauma illuminated why she repeatedly engaged in shoplifting, a behavior that induced fear and terror, as it engendered in her a rudimentary sense of self (Lanius et al., 2020). She notes:

"I started shoplifting when I was 5. I'd pretend to add the quarter my mother gave me to the collection plate, then sink it deep and hot into the pocket of my Sunday dress. On the long walk home, I'd pass a pharmacy where I'd steal a Clark Bar or a Milky Way, pantomime leaving the quarter for my coke and with a mix of terror and thrill leave the store, sugar happy and known to myself. . . . I shoplifted well into my adulthood, at great risk to me were I to be caught. . . . It was always confusing why I did this. It was so, so risky. I knew that. But I think the adrenaline organized me, rising it seemed from my belly through my brain, from the back to the front. I felt my feet; I knew my hands and fingers; I had eyes. I was agency. It lit me up. It was essential. At 5 and still at 50, I didn't exist to myself except as the artful dodger [pickpocket]. At these moments, I existed; all of me, in the act of stealing, *I* would 'come online.'"

Feeling Something Is Better than Feeling Nothing at All: The Compulsion to Repeat

Despite the terrorizing effects that far outlive the traumatic event, traumatized people may compulsively find themselves in situations reminiscent of the original trauma. While this may seem puzzling, it aligns with how survival brain connections from the periaqueductal gray to the DMN, as discussed above, may lead to the seeking of dangerous situations to evoke a sense of self that feels alive, even if only within the grips of terror. From toxic substances to toxic relationships, the pursuit of danger fosters extreme fluctuations in arousal that bring the individual to life once more; on the downside, it increases the probability of further harm. Reckless behaviors that are "thrill seeking" can include shoplifting, speeding, self-harm, substance use, disordered eating, or instigating conflict with others. Beyond the initial rush, a sense of powerlessness ensues where the traumatized individual is vulnerable to dangerous outcomes yet helplessly stuck in a vicious cycle of despair. This is especially prominent in cases of childhood trauma, where the absence of a safe caregiver or place for refuge can prime the DMN (Teicher et al., 2016) to only come online in the presence of threat. Critically, as the DMN is vital for social connection, the traumatized self may only be able to engage with another under conditions of threat.

The same trauma survivor quoted above elaborated further on the idea of seeking intensely arousing experiences to elicit a trauma response that, in effect, stimulates their periaqueductal gray to in turn reignite their DMN. Here, their sense of self became intimately linked to the periaqueductal gray–DMN connection such that the trauma response becomes the state in which they feel the most "alive." The predisposition and incentive to remain in a defensive state affects how they seek and define interactions with other people. They wrote:

"But there is always seeking of 'the other' embedded in this risk taking, and the wilder the need, the less discriminating who 'the other' is. It's not someone to stop you exactly, it's someone to meet you, to register you, to certify your existence. Shoplifting then not only provides the sense of self, it evokes the sense of [the] other."

Many theoretical models of personality have considered child–caregiver interactions as critical determinants for how an individual engages with the world. The child easily learns patterns of behaviors and internalizes them as "normal interactions," since they comprise their first memories. These interactions become habitual for the child and can be difficult to change, even if they are found to be maladaptive later in life (Briere, Kaltman, & Green, 2008; Briere & Runtz, 1990). Our biological maturation processes are strongly influenced by attachment responses, where modulation of physiological arousal is typically developed within the scaffolding of attunement from a consistent caregiver (Siegel, 2020; Yehuda et al., 2001, 2005). The synchrony felt with a familiar caregiver helps regulate the child in response to perceived danger and keeps the child within a contained zone of arousal, enveloping them in a felt sense of safety and nurturance. According to attachment theory (Ainsworth, 1978; Bowlby, 1979), a "safe base" plays a crucial role in biological development because it establishes cognitive schemas and the lens through which we see ourselves and the world, allowing us to contextualize new experiences through this framework. However, in the absence of a consistent or nurturing caregiver, children are left vulnerable to extreme fluctuations in arousal that are uncontained and overwhelming. This unbridled physiological and emotional distress leaves them destabilized without any safe base to depend upon.

For example, if a caregiver was inconsistent with their affection and the child was forced to endure a never-ending cycle of ambivalent presence followed by withdrawal or abuse, it can leave a child confused and searching for safety by any means necessary. This can manifest as anxious obedience to attain their caregiver's affection or extreme emotional numbing to close themselves off to an unpredictable and unsafe world. Children without a "safe base" may find it difficult to discern that abusive behavior is wrong, and may even feel deserving of it, causing extreme feelings of self-blame and shame (Briere, 1992; Briere & Elliott, 2003). These feelings can foster the development of deeply rooted beliefs, such as "I am bad" or "I don't deserve to feel anything positive." As such, it can be difficult to seek out or provide alternative feelings, such as love or affection, in future adult relationships, since there is no existing template for these feelings. The only template that exists, branded in the DMN, is for negative self-beliefs and devastating feelings. Consequently, traumatized individuals may often find that it is easier or more comfortable to reengage in abusive patterns rather than resist these patterns, leading to forms of behavioral reenactment that can manifest in revictimization patterns or harm to others. Here, the existence of the self may be dependent upon the periaqueductal gray's hijacking of the DMN (Lanius et al., 2020), perpetuating the role that terror plays in "feeling alive" and connecting to others.

Individuals stuck in patterns of revictimization may seek out stimulation in their environment that replicates the adverse emotional states experienced at the time of the trauma. In the aftermath of repeated childhood trauma, survivors may feel inclined to revert to adverse emotional states and may, in turn, become preoccupied with the trauma at the expense of fully experiencing life (Briere, 1992; Briere et al., 2024). In a sense, they continually re-create the terror of the past; for so long, it was their normal. For example, victims of sexual assault during childhood are more likely to be abused by their partners or strangers, thus subconsciously repeating the familiar cycle of the past. In addition, there is a higher prevalence of childhood sexual and emotional abuse among sex workers (Stoltz et al., 2007), where they may re-create familiar patterns of anxious obedience from childhood by trading sex for survival and use their trade to search for emotional intimacy from another human being (Herman, 2023). Richard Kluft (1990) described the grooming process of sex workers with the following quote:

> Beauty, yes. Sexual expertise, somewhat. That can be taught easier than you think. What is important above all is obedience. And how do you get obedience? You get women who have had sex with their fathers, their uncles, their brothers—you know, someone they love and fear and do not dare to defy. (p. 25)

It is critical to note that this vulnerability to coercive control stems from *below* conscious awareness, where the objectification and coinciding feelings of shame and worthlessness represent normalcy for the individual (Herman, 1992b). Here, the act of emotionally depraved sex itself, which was previously a traumatic experience, would activate the periaqueductal gray and reignite the DMN to bring online a semblance of existence for the self through "connection" with another. Seeking these experiences becomes primal, where continuous foraging for danger feeds the human need for connection. Here, feeling seen and wanted, and thus feeling alive, becomes coupled to the sexual experience, setting up a cycle for addiction. A cyclical negative state of withdrawal stems from the abandonment after the sexual act, which reinforces future desperation for the guise of intimacy afforded by these sexual acts. Victims of intimate partner violence are twice as likely to have experienced a childhood history of incest, where intimacy is linked to powerless submission. A history of incest strengthens the dynamic of being obedient to the perpetrator, reinforcing the cycle of abuse and the temporary state of reconciliation that follows. For the adult with a traumatized inner child, seeking this feeling of threat and danger is the only learned avenue for social connection. The individual may not stop or prevent the perpetrator from exerting their abusive behaviors in a frantic attempt to feel seen and wanted, which reinforces the schema through which they view themselves.

In a similar vein, adults who perpetrate abuse in their own family homes are more likely to have grown up in a turbulent or abusive environment themselves. A chronically abusive caregiving environment can foster feelings of defeat and learned helplessness among family members (Seligman, 1972), yielding adaptive responses in adulthood that can range from conditioned defeat to a hunger for power. It is possible that sensory and emotional deprivation as a child in the absence of a soothing caregiver may result in foundational sensory integrative and emotional regulatory capacities, giving rise to sensory processing challenges (over- or underresponsivity to sensory events) and/or stimulus-seeking behavior. Behaviorally, this may manifest in either withdrawal or aggression toward others. For those who tend toward aggression, they may be attracted to the rush they get from exerting control over others they had observed or experienced during their child-hood (Briere, 1988; Briere & Lanktree, 2011). Intense violence becomes the only means to avoid deeper feelings of powerlessness and defeat (Briere, Hodges, & Godbout, 2010). The scenes of violent "bonding" fulfill the attachment they crave from the victim. For the withdrawn individual, internalized distress may manifest as self-injurious in nature, from cutting to binge eating. Taken together, engage-ment in patterns of abuse ingrained during childhood allows for a re-created feel-ing of threat that may be critical to the traumatized sense of self. Feeling terrorized may be the easiest way to evoke the sense of the other, setting the stage for the compulsion to repeat the trauma. In extreme cases, reenactment may be the only way to fully remember the atrocities of the past and evoke the repressed self that is haunted by disintegrated traumatic memories.

Pierre Janet (1889) theorized that traumatic memories are the basis for the development of alternate states of consciousness, including dissociative fugue states or chronic states of helplessness or depression. He postulated that intrusive thoughts, nightmares, and flashbacks of traumatic events can be all consuming for the individual, and, in some cases, can stunt an individual's personality develop-ment. Fixation on these memories can lead to behavioral reenactment and, in turn, subconsciously drive individuals toward situations reminiscent of the original trauma. Sigmund Freud (1896) postulated similar sentiments in his work describ-ing hysterical symptoms, where he described patients who would "repeat repressed memories in their behavior rather than remember it as something belonging to the past" (p. 187). He went on to apply the term *repetition compulsion* to this phenomenon, where he explained that feelings that cannot be explicitly remem-bered or expressed in words would be manifested in actions. Loewald (1971) and Cohen (1980) hypothesized that compulsions to repeat traumatic events are owed to the ego's maladaptive integration of the memory into consciousness, which pre-cipitates posttraumatic stress symptoms of reliving traumatic experiences through flashbacks. The individual's worldview has been indelibly shaped by traumatic events, and they may only feel in control when they experience what's familiar. Unlearning maladaptive patterns requires extensive repetition of adaptive patterns to correct the deeply embedded template laid down during early experiences of being cared (or uncared) for. This process involves rewiring the DMN to foster the restoration of a self that is capable of embracing safety.

Sensorimotor Interventions

Sensorimotor psychotherapeutic approaches emphasize conscious attention to the body's postures, movements, and somatic (bodily) experiences. These approaches emphasize the importance of restoring a sense of agency through physical mastery over the environment, where the body's actions previously failed or betrayed one's intentions during a traumatic experience. This is hypothesized to result in sensory and motoric fragmentation, where individuals experience sensations and actions without any context, such as smelling a cologne previously worn by a perpetrator and hiding when hearing footsteps at the door, all the while feeling the presence of a looming threat. This sense of physical helplessness is thought to have reverberations upon one's sense of self, resulting in thoughts and beliefs that one is flawed, broken, or not to be trusted. Importantly, sensorimotor approaches center how traumatic memory traces may be evoked from incoming body-based stimuli. For example, an individual who was raped in a reclined position may experience intense anxiety and intrusive memories when having to assume that position again at the doctor's office given their previous experience of helplessness and terror.

Here, sensorimotor interventions facilitate the completion of actions that an individual could not carry out at the time of the trauma, which is hypothesized to help integrate the sensorimotor fragments of the memory into a coherent, past-centered narrative. Neurobiologically, this may result in a decoupling of the posterior DMN and sensorimotor network, which may then lead to the traumatic memory being remembered rather than relived. In the words of traumatized individuals who have experienced this phenomenon, one said, "Instead of the memory coming from a gaping wound, it is now coming from a projector in my mind," while the other said, "It's like you're allowing me to experience my painful memories in a safe space, and it kind of releases from my body and, afterward, I'm more able to look at it from a distance, instead of it being in my body."

Sensorimotor approaches focus on moving through alternative, more adaptive or self-protective postures or actions (discussed more in Chapter 9), such as pushing an exercise ball off the body while in a reclined or lying position, to restore a felt sense of the physical body as capable and powerful. Small-scale clinical trials have shown sensorimotor approaches, such as somatic trauma therapy (Rothschild, 2000, 2017), sensorimotor psychotherapy (Ogden, Pain, & Fisher, 2006), somatic experiencing (Brom et al., 2017; Levine, 2010), and sensory motor arousal regulation therapy (SMART; Warner, Koomar, Lary, & Cook, 2013), have been effective in improving arousal regulation and reducing PTSD symptoms (Classen et al., 2021; Finn, Warner, Price, & Spinazzola, 2018; Gene-Cos, Fisher, Ogden, & Cantrell, 2016; Kuhfuß, Maldei, Hetmanek, & Baumann, 2021; Langmuir, Kirsh, & Classen, 2012; Payne, Levine, & Crane-Godreau, 2015; Warner, Spinazzola, Westcott, Gunn, & Hodgdon, 2014). For the traumatized child, sensorimotor play is both a developmentally important occupation and a conduit to reorganizing survival brain-level circuitry (Goodyear-Brown, 2009; Warner et al., 2013). PLAY, one of the basic affects put forth by Panksepp (1998), is an innate drive emergent from the periaqueductal gray, alongside defensive fight/flight and shutdown responses. Utilizing PLAY as a therapeutic medium may thwart or replace ingrained defensive responses at this level of the survival brain. PLAY may allow us access to these deeper brain responses and help reorient the child's defenses toward seeking positive and safe social connections.

Children and Their Predisposition for Sensory Seeking

Trauma that occurs during or throughout childhood fundamentally interferes with the brain's and body's development. This points to a critical need to take a neurodevelopmental approach to treatment for children affected by trauma. From birth to age 7, children are highly motivated to move their bodies and engage in rich sensorimotor experiences, from pulling their bodies up against gravity to stand to mastering the monkey bars on the playground. Sensorimotor integration during this developmental period promotes mastery of the environment and engenders a sense of self that exists as a confidently separate entity in relation to the other. However, a child who has felt unsafe in their body and/or environment may lack the foundational sense of trust in themselves and others needed to meet their own needs and to navigate the world. For the child who has experienced conditions of prolonged threat, they may only come to understand and feel "normal" in defensive states, including hypervigilant high arousal states. High arousal states in children can be achieved through excessive engagement in alerting sensory experiences, such as spinning or climbing to dangerous heights. In a sense, the natural motivation to engage in sensorimotor play can be co-opted to develop a compulsive seeking of arousing sensations and an avoidance of calm interpersonal engagement. The child who experienced chronic inescapable traumatization and is prone to a dissociative shutdown defensive response may either seek excessive stimulation in an attempt to combat hypoarousal (and to feel "alive") or avoid sensorimotor play entirely to prevent experiencing any arousing sensations linked to a previously terrifying bodily state.

Regardless of the clinical presentation, developmental trauma fundamentally alters how the "self" is experienced; it is only online when in high arousal or danger, or it becomes coupled with a dissociated, protective yet withdrawn state. This necessitates a return to the foundations of sensory integrative opportunities with the attuned presence of a co-regulatory adult as early as possible to prevent trauma-related alterations becoming baked into one's neurodevelopmental wiring within critical periods of development.

Lola from Chapter 4 sought an excessive amount of movement and climbing to the extent that she endangered her physical safety. From a neurodevelopmental standpoint, Lola never experienced sensory co-regulation in the form of being held and rocked with a reliable caregiver—instead, she experienced abuse and neglect during her formative infant and toddler years. From her earliest days, Lola's nervous system and brain adapted to both anticipate threat and shut off her emotions of despair when her survival needs were not met. Her steady state became one of hyperarousal, which overflowed into her body given her lack of motor inhibition at her developmental stage. Post- (or peri-) traumatic symptoms often appear as physical restlessness, impulsivity, and poor attention in childhood, given the cortex's lack of maturity to properly inhibit or dampen the physical urges tied to overwhelming emotions. Lola's body often seemed confused; she was seeking regulating movement and input into her muscles in a desperate attempt to expunge her excess arousal, but her seeking of this input was disorganized, inappropriate, and unsafe. Furthermore, the feeling of danger is a state in which Lola felt most at home. She could not relate to her calm adoptive parents telling her to stop and be careful. No one had been calming or careful with her body when she had needed it most in her early years.

Once Lola began occupational therapy, she required substantial scaffolding to meet her high thresholds for movement and climbing in order to achieve her preferred arousal state, albeit in a safe and organized manner. Each day, Lola climbed to the top of a play structure and onto cabinets to get her preferred toys. At first, Lola resisted any assistance or safety rules as a knee-jerk response to the imposed control, but the therapist (after first verbally alerting her that she would need to physically help her to keep her safe) consistently and gently helped her body out of precarious situations. Over time, Lola became more accepting of these consistent and firm safety "rules" as she came to realize that the therapist's predictability and reliability felt good, and the physical assistance provided her with the somatic sensory input needed to begin to safely sense her physical boundaries. Lola's therapist continued to attune to her arousal needs; high swinging and jumping onto soft pillows, climbing to the ceiling in a safety harness, and running and crashing her body into a pile of soft blocks repeatedly allowed her to meet her sensory thresholds while her therapist kept her organized. Over time, Lola was able to let down her guard as she recognized her therapist as someone who could understand her thirst for high-arousal play and simultaneously engender feelings of safety.

One day, Lola climbed to the top of the play structure as was customary, but for the first time, she asked her therapist to carry her down. Her therapist enveloped her body with the touch and gravitational support Lola craved but was previously too fearful to allow. Without this primal experience in her early history, Lola was unable to exist in the world without exerting a large amount of control over others. Here, Lola experienced her body being held by a safe adult, and she was able to surrender gravitational control without spinning into a state of terror. This initial relinquishing of control was necessary to develop a deep sense of trust in another while in a vulnerable state, which was a prerequisite to developing a better sense of control over her own bodily states. This breakthrough moment was just one of many to come, as Lola became less combative with her therapist, teachers, and parents who began joining her sessions to learn how to gain her body's trust.

Shame and Moral Injury as Threats to the Self

A moral injury may develop when a deeply held moral code has been violated, which has been associated with manifestations of PTSD, depression, and suicidal ideation (Drescher et al., 2011; Jinkerson, 2016; Litz et al., 2009). Moral injury can have a profound effect on an individual's sense of self and identity as well as their relations with others; a Vietnam veteran once noted, "I cannot look anyone in the eye for fear that they will see the stain on my soul" (Frewen & Lanius, 2015, p. 297). Terpou and colleagues (2022) and Kearney, Terpou, and colleagues (2023) examined the brain correlates of the DMN and sensorimotor network during recall of a morally injurious event among individuals with and without PTSD. Remembering a morally injurious event was associated with stronger connectivity between the periaqueductal gray and the DMN (Terpou et al., 2022), as well as between the posterior DMN and sensorimotor network (Kearney, Terpou, et al., 2023) in PTSD. Here, individuals with moral injury-related PTSD may predominantly view themselves through the stained, cracked lens of their moral injury. Thus, recollection of the event evokes intense visceral and somatic (muscle tension, pain, heat) sensations and arousal, tainting their sense of self and identity.

Additionally, moral injury has been associated with increased neural activation of the insula, a reflective brain region that encodes visceral sensations (Lloyd et al., 2021). Importantly, the posterior insula receives raw interoceptive information from the brainstem that represents the bodily self (Craig, 2009; Namkung, Kim, & Sawa, 2017; Uddin, Nomi, Hebert-Seropian, Ghaziri, & Boucher, 2017). Examples of raw interoceptive information include pain, feeling a sinking pit in the stomach, and nausea, as well as the shuddering experienced from moral disgust (Stephani, Fernandez-Baca Vaca, Maciunas, Koubeissi, & Luders, 2011; Ying et al., 2018). Thus, increased activation of the posterior insula during moral injury memory recall may represent an insult to the somatic or visceral aspect of the sense of self. For example, while recalling morally injurious events, some individuals described feeling pain and nausea, "an internal gnawing sensation," and feeling as though they were "being eaten up inside" (Lloyd et al., 2021). Taken together, these somatic sensations may directly inform self-related perspectives, the sense of self, and identity in the context of moral injury and psychological trauma.

Going forward, it will be critical to develop neuroscientifically guided treatments that can facilitate the healing of traumatic insults to the self. Treatments that work to regulate the visceral sensations and arousal associated with activation of the periaqueductal gray and the posterior insula, as experienced during moral injury recall, and to decouple the periaqueductal gray and sensorimotor network from the individual's sense of self and its related memories are crucial. Such treatments likely intervene at the level of the survival brain, which can then transform how we perceive ourselves and the world through bottom-up regulation of the DMN (see Bridging to Practice 8 for additional guidance about how to implement these strategies in a therapeutic setting). The sole use of cognitive interventions without attention to deep structures, such as the periaqueductal gray, that underpin the visceral experience of moral injury recall may improve an individual's ability to *know*, rationally, that it was not their fault, but it will not relieve the guttural sensations associated with *feeling* that it was. Furthermore, overlooking the involvement of sensorimotor processing in traumatic memory may lead to plateaus in trauma processing, where intervening only at the level of voluntary thought and behavior can lead to an impasse where the somatic manifestations of trauma live on. To fully transform the sense of self and become firmly grounded in one's identity, visceral and somatic sensations must align with narratives about who one is in the world. The neuroplasticity behind this transformation may involve the attenuation of survival brain responses and restoration of healthy DMN functioning in the aftermath of trauma.

**CASE EXAMPLE: Building on Shaky Ground—
The Use of Cognitive Processing Therapy after Moral Injury**

Joanne is a 35-year-old woman who worked as a journalist for her local news station in the United Kingdom. She often reported from the field and covered a broad spectrum of events, from food festivals to horrific car accidents. Each gruesome news story seemed to leave an indelible imprint on her, making it more difficult to rebound each time. Her sleep and mood became more and more negatively affected by her job. She continued to manage until she was faced with the most terrifying news event of her career. Joanne was called to work early one morning to cover a gruesome series of stabbings that left a family murdered, including both parents and their two young children. As the news coverage and investigation unfolded, it appeared that it was a hate crime. As a member of the local community, Joanne was devastated. However, she felt a civic duty to report the news regardless of how broken she felt. For a 2-week period, she was covering the event nearly 24/7, publishing news articles in the press every day, and operating with little to no sleep. Each article written would recap the event and article of the previous day, forcing her to relive the terror and gut-wrenching feelings over again, each day. She forced herself to compartmentalize her anger and profound sadness when writing about the innocent children whose lives were taken away. At the same time, her news coverage of this event was gaining national acclaim, and she was starting to become recognized positively for her contributions and humanity while reporting on the event. Joanne described feeling "dirty" and guilt ridden when hearing this praise because she felt that it was at the expense of this horrific tragedy. After the news cycle for this event died down, Joanne's view of the world was left shattered, and she had difficulty focusing, sleeping, or even being around other people. She described the event as the "straw that broke the camel's back." A few months later, she had to take a leave of absence from work to deal with her trauma symptoms.

Approximately 1 year later, Joanne went to see a psychologist to help address her difficulties coping with the aftermath of this morally injurious event. She underwent a course of cognitive processing therapy, where she was able to identify the negative beliefs that she came to hold so firmly. First, she wrote an impact statement about how the event affected her self-esteem and shaped how she viewed the world, particularly in relation to the themes of safety and trust. In particular, Joanne struggled with a deep sense that the national acclaim she received for her journalism was at odds with her own moral compass, which felt completely broken. Since Joanne's view of her community and the world at large was shattered, she felt that she no longer knew herself, as she often felt raw emotions, like panic, rage, and fear, take over. The psychologist helped her identify "stuck points," which are thoughts about one's own self or the world following a traumatic experience that may be indicative of how one feels but may not necessarily be wholly true and can pose as barriers for recovery. For example, Joanne held the belief that she was dirty for being a vessel that the media used to sensationalize news events. The psychologist helped her to challenge this belief and reframe this thought toward a more balanced perspective to alleviate some of the guilt she felt. She was able to shift her thoughts and tell herself that although she could not control how the news cycle worked, she still made the effort to maintain her own code of morality because she always kept the innocent people lost in this tragedy at the forefront of her mind. Overall, cognitive processing therapy helped her to become much more aware of the connection between her thoughts and trauma-related emotions, such as guilt, anger, and shame. Subsequently, she became much less avoidant of her thoughts and felt she could let them come to the surface more.

However, about 10 months after completing this therapy, her trauma symptoms reemerged when she was triggered by a similar news event. Joanne felt her mood shift and had renewed feelings of anger and guilt. Due to cognitive processing therapy, Joanne was able to identify her emotions much more readily and figure out why she was triggered, which stopped her from spiraling into a deeper hole of negative emotions. She knew that the intensity of her emotions was becoming increasingly difficult to manage and realized that she needed help regulating the raw emotions that were threatening to regain control. This time, she sought out different treatments that could specifically help her focus on reducing the negative raw affect, including DBR and EMDR therapy. These approaches focused on regulating her visceral and emotional responses, and in turn helped to reinforce the alternative thinking strategies she learned through cognitive processing therapy.

Changing the Sense of Self through Psychedelic-Assisted Psychotherapy: Coming into View

Psychedelics have been shown to have a significant effect on the functioning of the DMN (Carhart-Harris et al., 2014; Gattuso et al., 2023). By disrupting the typical activity of the DMN, these substances can facilitate profound changes in perception, cognition, and emotional state, opening up new avenues for therapeutic intervention. Psychedelic-assisted psychotherapy typically comprises multiple phases, starting with a preparation session where the therapist and client prepare for potential occurrences while they are administered the psychedelic (Mithoefer, Grob, & Brewerton, 2016). The next session focuses on administration of the psychedelic substance and typically involves two therapists who support the client throughout the session and allow the psychedelic journey to naturally evolve. Following the psychedelic session, the integration sessions are critical for assimilating the material that emerged during the psychedelic session, which can take up to several months to process. Upon completion of this therapy, many individuals frequently report a profound change in how they perceive themselves and the world, as described in the case below.

CASE EXAMPLE: Marie and MDMA-Assisted Psychotherapy

Marie is a 64-year-old woman who grew up with a mother who frequently told her that she wished Marie had never been born. Her father was largely absent. Marie learned early on in her life that the best way to survive was to hide. Being seen, especially by her mother, was frequently met with rejection and hostility. Being invisible therefore became an essential means of survival for Marie. Despite Marie's difficult home life, she excelled at school. She was particularly talented in English, and creative writing was an important outlet for her to express her inner emotional turmoil. Marie often expressed how she was permeated by feelings of shame that left her feeling like she was an abhorrent human nondeserving of love and affection. These feelings predominated most of Marie's life.

In her early 60s, Marie began reading about psychedelic-assisted psychotherapy. This piqued her interest because, despite years of helpful psychotherapy, she had never been able to resolve the intense feelings of shame that permeated her life. Marie therefore began a course of MDMA (ecstasy)-assisted psychotherapy. Marie had a profound revelation during this treatment. During the psychedelic session, Marie described being welcomed into a world by a motherly figure. For the first time, she experienced profound love and compassion from this presence. Marie initially felt quite overwhelmed by the enormous love and compassion emanating from this figure. However, over time, Marie described feeling more and more held by the love and compassion that she experienced. During the following integration sessions, Marie became increasingly aware that her feelings of badness were slowly fading, and she began to notice an emerging feeling of self-compassion. At first, this was rather startling for her, but through guidance from her therapist, she was able to embrace a life that was no longer pervaded by shame. Over time, this allowed Marie to feel deserving of being seen and begin tolerating the support and connection from individuals around her.

Restoring the Sense of Self and Identity: Toward Increased Malleability of the Self

Emerging evidence indeed points toward malleability of the DMN in response to treatment (King et al., 2016; Kluetsch et al., 2014; Nicholson et al., 2016, 2018, 2020), which speaks to the brain's capacity to heal after trauma. King and colleagues have shown that connectivity within the DMN can be changed in response to treatment with mindfulness-based meditation in veterans with PTSD. Specifically, connectivity between the posterior node of the DMN increased with the anterior node of the DMN in response to fearful faces, which the authors attributed to greater engagement with threat cues in individuals with PTSD after mindfulness training.

Moreover, neurofeedback has been shown to normalize decreased connectivity within the DMN in PTSD (Kluetsch et al., 2014; Nicholson et al., 2018, 2020). Neurofeedback is a form of biofeedback, which uses a brain computer interface to provide feedback about brain functioning. Here, individuals can learn to change patterns of brain activity and associated distress through ongoing feedback on a computer screen. Alpha-rhythm neurofeedback has been shown to normalize functioning of the DMN as well as reduce the chance of being diagnosed with PTSD. Indeed, in a recent randomized controlled trial of alpha-based neurofeedback in PTSD, 20 weekly sessions of neurofeedback led to remission rates and symptom reduction effect sizes that are in line with current gold-standard treatment interventions for PTSD (Nicholson et al., 2020). Importantly, in this study, PTSD symptoms continued to improve at the 3-month follow-up and there were no patient dropouts in the trial, which speaks to the tolerability of this intervention. Furthermore, emerging evidence also points to neurofeedback being able to target deep brain structures, including the periaqueductal gray (Nicholson et al., 2016), a survival brain structure that is associated with trauma-related visceral sensations and arousal that has been shown to drive self-related perspectives mediated by the DMN in PTSD under threat, as described above. We suggest that neurofeedback may therefore be an important adjunctive intervention targeting altered self-perception and identity by restoring the connectivity of DMN and thus aid in the restoration of the self in the aftermath of trauma.

CASE EXAMPLE: Emily, Overcoming the Intergenerational Transmission of Trauma in an Indian Residential School Survivor

By Patricia Vickers, PhD

On the northwest coast of British Columbia, Indigenous nations have a celebration of the passing on of history, relationships, and transactions through a potlatch or feast. The hosting tribe provides the meal and gifts to all who choose to witness the transaction. Traditional names, histories, and connections are all affirmed and grounded in protocol and process. Our ancestral laws are the foundation for all relationships and have never been extinguished. This is our primary resource for healing and wellness.

Regardless of where we reside, we have a lived knowledge of our current social statistics[1] and understand the impact of Indian residential schools (IRSs) as the primary contributing factor to intergenerational trauma in our personal lives and the lives of all our relations.

The case example, named Emily, is a 52-year-old Indigenous woman who was married with two adult children. Emily received alpha-rhythm 30 EEG neurofeedback sessions, each lasting 20 minutes, and the protocol and process followed ancestral law. Clinical assistance was provided if the client requested DBR due to dysregulation from childhood memories arising when their brain was sustaining an alpha state.

During the assessment, I (Dr. Vickers) asked Emily if she was living with PTSD, and she was not certain. It was suggested that as a second-generation IRS survivor (her parents attended IRSs), she would likely be living with PTSD. I read her the symptoms of PTSD for informed consent, and she agreed.

After completing her eighth session, Emily became aware that she has an exaggerated startle response. Without prompting, she began to speak about the abuse that took place in the IRS and its consequences on her family life while growing up.

When Emily came in for her 13th session, she noticed how she is "not stressed when plans aren't able to be carried through." She also mentioned a dream that she had between her neurofeedback sessions. She said, "I was in my home in an empty room that had see-through curtains. Everyone outside could see inside the house. There was a room next to the empty room that was dark inside, and I was afraid to open the door to go into the room." She asked me what I thought her dream meant, and I answered that perhaps her brain wanted to release a memory that frightened her; she agreed. Through tears, she disclosed in her 14th session that her father had thrown her infant brother against the wall in a drunken rage, which resulted in a traumatic brain injury. In her recount of the memory, she was clear and calm while expressing the pain of the horror. She went on to say that she understood her father's rage and that it was a result of the violence that he both witnessed and experienced in his IRS. She concluded with the statement that she loved and forgave her father for his violence.

Emily's personal process throughout neurofeedback remarkably moved from recalling the horrifying memory, to understanding the impact of her father's history on his behavior toward his family, to forgiveness, all within days. She noted that neurofeedback accelerated her healing process in a calming way.

---

[1] Available at *www150.statcan.gc.ca/n1/pub/41-20-0002/412000022023004-eng.htm*.

Within a month, Emily recounted two horrifying memories and integrated them into her present-day life, expressing how the traumatic experiences were "covered" in her interior self and how recalling them brought understanding to the horror and terror she had lived with for over 40 years.

In conclusion, Emily not only experienced rapid healing from a horrific memory but she also understood that the violence was related to the intergenerational transmission of trauma inflicted on her family by IRSs. She spoke at an evening dinner gathering among a group of 22 individuals who had received neurofeedback therapy. Here, Emily spoke to the violence that she witnessed as a child, how it impacted her, and that she did not blame her parents. Her courage inspired everyone that evening. Regarding interconnectedness, compassionate understanding, and the power of ancestral teachings, IRS attendee and Secwépemc elder Dave Belleau eloquently summarized the connection with ancestors and one another. Dave recounts asking one of his fellow students, "How in the hell he survived the whipping (with the priest's belt, buckle end on his back) when he was just a little guy." Dave states that his friend answered, "I survived by seeing the feet of all of you other children standing around the bed and knowing I was not alone."

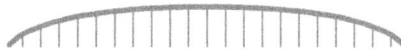

BRIDGING TO PRACTICE 8
Engaging in Reckless Behaviors to Feel Alive

In many cases, clients find themselves repeatedly involved in risky behaviors like extreme sports, substance use (most commonly stimulants), conflicts, self-harm, and theft. These actions are often labeled as "bad," and clients are urged to cease them. However, the underlying reasons for these behaviors are often overlooked and not thoroughly examined. These behaviors commonly stem from intense emotional numbness, which is associated with a lack of feeling fully alive. Exploring the potential link between risky behaviors and seeking a sense of aliveness is crucial.

Risky behaviors are typically accompanied by heightened arousal and an adrenaline rush, which helps counter the emotional numbness and creates a sensation of being alive. Understanding the motivations behind these behaviors can not only reduce the shame associated with them but also foster a deeper understanding of why clients engage in such actions. With increasing emotional awareness, clients often realize that they turn to substances, provoke conflicts, self-harm, or steal in a bid to feel alive amidst emotional numbness. This feeling of aliveness appears accessible only during moments of intense arousal for individuals experiencing profound emotional anesthesia.

Questions to ask your client:

1. Do you ever feel emotionally numb?
2. Does it feel like you are not fully alive?
3. Have you ever participated in risky activities? For example, have you engaged in extreme sports? What about using substances, particularly stimulants like amphetamines, cocaine, or crystal meth? Have you ever found yourself in conflicts, engaged in self-harm, or resorted to stealing?
4. What happens when you engage in these behaviors? Do they affect how emotionally numb you feel? Do they affect your level of feeling alive?
5. Do you think you may be engaging in these behaviors to feel more alive?

Once you have confirmed that your client resorts to reckless actions to seek a sense of aliveness, it is crucial to pinpoint behaviors that can provide an adrenaline rush without posing a risk. For instance, engaging in high-intensity exercise, viewing awe-inspiring nature images or videos, taking a cold shower, or listening to energizing music can be beneficial. Gradually, it is important to monitor the physical states that trigger reckless behaviors (refer to Chapter 7) and substitute them with safer activities that can elevate arousal levels and trigger a safe adrenaline surge.

9

Becoming Whole

SYNCHRONIZING THE MIND, BRAIN, AND BODY

Nothing is created or destroyed, only transformed.
—ANTOINE LAVOISIER (1789)

Throughout this book, we have emphasized the remarkable adaptability of the brain, mind, and body in response to chronic, inescapable threat posed by trauma. Importantly, many brain regions and circuits affected by trauma, especially in the survival section of the brain, are inaccessible to language, thus posing challenges for traditional psychotherapeutic methods relying on language as the primary means of action. A critical adaptation to trauma also involves the brain–body disconnect, where traumatized individuals can no longer optimally regulate their bodily distress through top-down brain control mechanisms. This leaves the traumatized individual with the agony that gnaws at the core of their being, frequently leaving them feeling shattered and hollow inside. Critically, their bodily dysregulation and feelings of unsafety frequently cannot be fully soothed through verbal psychotherapy that targets primarily thoughts or beliefs. Feelings of safety remain an unknown concept for many traumatized persons, especially for those who have experienced repeated trauma from an early age. The brain, mind, and body have yet to adapt to these unfamiliar sensations.

However, through the power of neuroplasticity, feelings of security can become a known entity after trauma. Through the therapeutic process, a sense of safety can gradually establish itself as the brain's new baseline, leading to a renewed sense of existence and belonging in the world. Navigating this frequently challenging journey requires careful consideration, ensuring that each step taken nurtures a feeling of safety and stability within the individual. Embracing "the slower you go, the faster you get there" (Kluft, 1990) underscores the importance of permitting progress to unfold at a pace that feels safe to the traumatized individual. Here, employing the metaphor of allowing a larva to metamorphose into a butterfly at its natural pace can provide a beacon of hope. Within this chapter, we delve further into a myriad of bottom-up and top-down therapeutic approaches that act as pathways for neuroplasticity, facilitating healing by fostering a sense of safety within oneself, in relationships, and in community. Ultimately, these approaches can be intricately interwoven to facilitate a reunion of brain, mind, and body and the restoration of the self within community.

Bridging the Three Sections of the Brain: Bottom-Up and Top-Down Approaches

Bottom-Up Approaches

From a bottom-up neurobiological vantage point, we begin to untangle the mystery of how trauma may be stored "in the body" (Rothschild, 2000, 2017; van der Kolk, 2014). Here, we explore therapeutic approaches that operate from this subcortically driven perspective and hinge on the idea that incoming sensations can influence higher-order cognition. As mentioned throughout this book, the integration of raw sensory input with raw affect at the level of the survival brain may be disrupted and/or not fully transmitted to the cortex, resulting in a cascading effect on executive functioning, modulation of affective and motivational states, and conscious awareness of physical bodily experiences. Bottom-up dominant approaches may be particularly beneficial for individuals who feel numb or otherwise disconnected from their bodies, as no amount of talking will target the experience of no longer feeling fully alive. This is often true of those with a history of early attachment disruption and/or early childhood traumatization due to the overlap with robust sensorimotor development during childhood and adolescence (Perry, 2019), with the most critical developmental window occurring during the first 8 years of life (Lane et al., 2019).

Jean Ayres (1972), occupational therapist and pioneer of sensory integration theory, emphasized that active, motivated, sensory-rich engagement of the client in any therapeutic process is the key ingredient for promoting neuroplasticity, viewing the brain as a self-organizing system. This approach fosters a sense of self-mastery, where a consistent and satisfying ability to produce meaningful goal-directed action engenders a deep sense of trust and, thus, calm in the body and its interactions with the external world. We review bottom-up predominant psychotherapeutic approaches in turn. Importantly, we use the word *predominant*, as all these approaches inherently incorporate top-down processing by encouraging increased awareness and conscious attention to the lower happenings of the brain and body.

Sensorimotor psychotherapy (Fisher & Ogden, 2009; Ogden et al., 2006) involves active movements that address defensive posturing. Mindful attention to sensations, postures, and movements facilitates a reconnection of the body and sub-cortical processing to cortical awareness (Fisher, 2017). In a similar vein, somatic experiencing (Levine, 2010) pays special attention to the body's instinctual drive to bring previously thwarted or incomplete actions during traumatic events to completion to rewrite the body's story from perceived failure to success. SMART (Warner et al., 2014) incorporates elements from Ayres's (1972) sensory integrative approach and sensorimotor psychotherapy to emphasize lower-level vestibular and sensorimotor processing in the context of embodied trauma processing. These approaches center a mindful attentiveness to incoming sensorimotor information gleaned both from action and feedback from action, while recognizing that dysregulated arousal precludes one's ability to access higher-order cognition and language. Small-size clinical trials studying these approaches have shown promising results for reductions in PTSD symptoms and improvements in arousal regulation (Classen et al., 2021; Finn et al., 2018; Gene-Cos et al., 2016; Kuhfuß et al., 2021; Langmuir et al., 2012).

DBR (Corrigan & Christie-Sands, 2020; Corrigan, Young & Christie-Sands, 2024; Kearney, Corrigan, et al., 2023) also takes a neuroanatomically informed approach to understanding early sensorimotor mechanisms that transpire within a traumatic event. DBR emphasizes the key roles of the brainstem and midbrain in orienting an individual to a salient, potentially threatening stimulus and in exerting a "shock" response that is felt in the body before emotional processing occurs. Through attention to vestibular- and somatosensory-derived muscular tension from the orienting response, this approach also incorporates top-down processing to mindfully slow down and reorient the individual to their body in the present moment. Results from a randomized controlled trial of DBR show significant reductions in PTSD symptoms across all symptom clusters (reexperiencing, avoidance, negative alterations in cognitions and mood, alterations in arousal; Kearney, Corrigan, et al., 2023).

Other bottom-up approaches include the following:

- Equine-facilitated/equine-assisted psychotherapy (Lentini & Knox, 2015; McCullough, Risley-Curtiss, & Rorke, 2015; Naste et al., 2018; Palomar-Ciria & Bello, 2023) focuses on a therapeutic alliance with a horse, emphasizing the sense of connection to self and other and agency gained through touch, balance, and postural control.
- Trauma-sensitive yoga (Emerson & Hopper, 2011; Zaccari, Sherman, Higgins, & Kelly, 2024) focuses on guiding clients in tolerating titrated somatic sensation during yogic movements in a trauma-informed setting.
- Expressive arts therapy (Malchiodi, 2020, 2022; Schouten, de Niet, Knipscheer, Kleber, & Hutschemaekers, 2015), including theater, music, art, writing, and dance, taps into individuals' sense of agency by incorporating the physical body in meaningful, goal-oriented actions and expressions. Active engagement in artistic expression can be grounding for traumatized

individuals, allowing for the regulation of arousal, gradual toleration of trauma-related sensations and emotions, and integration of past traumas into a coherent self-referential story, as you will see in a case example below.

Encouraging individuals to reconnect with their felt bodily experiences within a positively valenced therapeutic alliance contradicts previous negatively valenced multisensory experiences and attachment disruptions. It is crucial to note that "bottom-up" approaches are not unidirectional; reconstructing the bridge between sensorial affect and cortical processing necessitates attention to top-down processes as well. Mindful attention to somatic experience may activate the medial prefrontal cortex (mPFC), known to be engaged in mindfulness-based approaches (Farb, Segal, & Anderson, 2013; Frewen et al., 2010; Ives-Deliperi, Solms, & Meintjes, 2011). The mPFC then down-regulates the lower regions involved in emotionality, arousal, and affect regulation.

Initially, the therapist acts as an externalized mPFC, attending to alterations in posture, arousal, and movements until the client can independently take notice. The client is then empowered to attend to, appreciate, and better regulate their affective and physiological defensive responses, restoring a sense of agency and trust in the body that begins to allow them to start embracing safe sensations. Utilizing somatic sensory input within a mindfulness framework, where individuals are guided in noticing the presence, intensity, and quality of stimulation, may bridge the brain–body disconnect that is often challenging to address in cognitive therapies. Individualized trauma-sensitive approaches enriched with somatic sensory input may support emotional and physiological regulation, foster safety within the therapeutic alliance, and facilitate the tolerance and integration of traumatic memories during psychotherapy sessions.

CASE EXAMPLE: Expressive Arts Therapy—Restoration through Community

By Cathy Malchiodi

When most practitioners hear the phrase "expressive arts therapy," they often imagine a series of activities, such as singing, drawing, or role play. These experiences may all be part of an expressive arts session, but as a form of psychotherapy this approach is much more than an art project or relaxation. It is an integrative method that is sensory based and action oriented—like other forms of psychotherapy, it includes enhancing the communication of feelings and expanding awareness of self. In contrast to most talk therapy, expressive arts therapy applies "bottom-up" strategies that start with movement, gesture, enactment, sound making, drawing, and playfulness to provide novel opportunities for expression that bypass language, or in some cases, stimulate narratives (Malchiodi, 2022). It is based on the idea that all stories begin as implicit (nonverbal or sensory based) experiences before becoming explicit (narratives; Damasio, 1998).

Expressive arts therapy is particularly well suited to supporting what we call "restorative relationships." In other words, it capitalizes on interaction through arts-based experiences to support synchrony, entrainment, attachment, and attunement between individuals. In a psychotherapy session, these relational moments occur between the therapist and individual, but expressive approaches are also particularly powerful in enhancing relationships and a sense of community within groups and families (Malchiodi, 2020). The sensory and implicit nature of these action-oriented experiences opens novel channels of communication when words may not be available because of traumatic stress or other challenges.

CASE EXAMPLE: Jacob—Reunification with Family and Self

A large part of my (Dr. Malchiodi) work as a psychotherapist has been in providing individual and group expressive arts therapy to active military and their families. Typically, this begins within the context of what are commonly referred to as "reintegration programs" where active military returning from duties abroad are reunited with their families through formalized workshops and events. These are usually intensive experiences at locations where large numbers of families are present and participate in a daily schedule of communal meals, couples' activities, and children's programming.

In these settings I generally first work with the soldier's children, introducing arts and play-based expression as a way to support their communication of their experiences as part of a military family. Initiating ways for these children to express the very real fears and terrors they have about their parents' exposure to life-threatening situations is one focus of these sessions. However, my primary goal is ultimately to enhance connection between family members and build community. The narratives that emerge from arts and play are expressions that parents are eventually invited to see, hear, and witness what their children are thinking and feeling through drawings, enactments, and storytelling. This is congruent with the core goal of reintegration programming: strengthening connection, attachment, and attunement to build resilience in the family system.

Jacob, an army lieutenant, attended a reintegration weekend with his wife and two children and peers he served with overseas. He had just returned to the United States after 6 months of service in the Middle East. It was not his first assignment to that region; he was deployed to both Iraq and Afghanistan, where he was in active combat for several years. According to the psychiatrist who previously worked with Jacob, he struggled with traumatic stress in the form of angry outbursts, insomnia, and hyperactivation when back in the United States and his wife and children were frequently exposed to his reactions. In particular, his relationship with his wife was strained and she reported to the psychiatrist that "Jacob is simply unavailable. I don't know what he is feeling because he refuses to talk about anything."

During one of the reintegration group sessions for school-age children, Jacob's 9-year-old son, Taylor, shared a story that deepened my understanding of his father's struggles. One experiential the children enthusiastically respond to in these sessions is creating a "safe place" for a rubber duck. I have on hand a variety of construction materials, colorful feathers, collage, and other art materials for each child to build a safe, peaceful, or soothing environment for the rubber duck. From an expressive arts perspective we are starting from a "somatosensory" place, pretending we are ducks through sound, movement, and play; experimenting and exploring the sensory qualities of art materials; and eventually creating a tangible expression that stimulates storytelling. While the children experience a sense of joy, playfulness, self-agency, and mastery in the process, the actual storytelling is consistently revealing.

In the case of children from military families, the stories that emerge about the duck and its "safe place" are most often about not only the child but also the soldier parent. Like many of his peers, Taylor built an elaborate safe structure for his "Colonel Duck," a duck that he explained was in charge of other ducks and led many dangerous missions. As he told me the story, Taylor emphasized that Colonel Duck often shouted at the other ducks and that he "spent a long time alone. He didn't want to play games or go to parties or have any fun." Taylor's observations obviously were consistent with the angry outbursts and withdrawal reported by Jacob's psychiatrist. But what was most intriguing and curious to me in Taylor's narrative were his last two comments: "He [Colonel Duck] feels really bad about having to kill people. He can't look at other people because he is so sad."

As part of the expressive arts therapy programming, I invite parents to community sessions where they can learn more about their children's participation. I also invite the children to share their art expressions and stories with their parents. Without any prompting, Taylor asked to read his story to his parents. Jacob quietly listened, with one visible tear rolling down his cheek. Both parents remained silent but clearly were emotional when Taylor spoke with conviction that his duck "can't look at other people because he is so sad."

It was soon after this parent–child session that Jacob contacted me for individual psychotherapy. In our initial meetings, we explored and worked through Jacob's concern for Taylor's obvious worries about his father, military deployment, and his stressful relationship with his wife. I supported him in discovering sensory-based ways through movement, sound, and image making to regulate mood swings, particularly anger and hyperactivation. Establishing a foundation for regulation in body and mind helped Jacob to begin to slowly examine more about his inability to be intimate with his wife and his feelings of frustration at not being a "good father" to Taylor and his younger daughter.

What we eventually learned through subsequent individual sessions was not surprising, but ultimately transformative for Jacob. In one session, Jacob explored his sensations about "combat" with a body outline using colors, shapes, and lines, as well as some simple gestures and poses through movement. While he expressed many different sensations of stress, pain, anger, and even fear through his movements and drawing, the most startling feature he included on his body outline was what he called "blindfolded eyes." When I asked him if he could tell me a little more about that feature on the outline, he said,

"You know, I have never been blindfolded like this person (referring to the body outline). But my biggest problem right now is I can't make eye contact. I can't make eye contact with my wife or Taylor or my young daughter. I am ashamed as a husband and a parent."

Jacob began in this moment to reveal an experience common to many soldiers who have been in active combat: moral injury. He was suffering with intense shame because he felt he had violated his own moral compass during his military service and actions he took as a soldier during combat. In the weeks following this session, Jacob's feelings of self-violation became the focus of expressive and sensory-based work, an example of self-restoration that is too detailed to present in this brief case description.

Reentry into community is not simple when traumatic stress in the form of hyperactivation and the shame of moral injury are present. Like Jacob, rejoining the community, whether it is reintegration with one's peers or with family, is circuitous. In this case, Jacob's longer process of reintegration with both community (military duties and peers) and family began after experiencing how Taylor interpreted his father's trauma reactions through art and story. Taylor's Colonel Duck's safe place and his narrative about a duck that "can't look at people" clearly communicated not only his father's traumatic stress but also the weight of moral injury that resulted in anger, sadness, and avoidance of intimacy. This was a significant turning point and became a way for Jacob to risk reaching out for help for his unresolved challenges. It was the beginning of repairing relationships with his wife and family and a restorative return to the military community.

Top-Down Approaches

From a top-down perspective, trauma-based treatment approaches focus on addressing the psychological and cognitive aspects of trauma by targeting higher brain functions, such as aspects of cognition, emotion regulation, and contextualizing the environment and surroundings. In part, these approaches can be considered an extension that can build on the bottom-up approaches discussed above, which formulate the emotional bedrock that can maximize the effect of top-down approaches. Top-down approaches aim to help individuals reprocess and integrate traumatic memories through identifying and reframing beliefs developed in the aftermath of trauma.

One such approach that has been often used as a frontline treatment for trauma is cognitive processing therapy (Resick et al., 2017; Resick, Monson, & Chard, 2024), which is a type of cognitive-behavioral therapy specifically designed to help individuals challenge and reframe distorted beliefs and thoughts related to the traumatic experience, promoting cognitive restructuring. The goal is to provide psychoeducation about PTSD to understand how trauma-related beliefs are created and challenge these beliefs to consider new and more balanced perspectives to reduce emotional distress. While cognitive processing therapy is helpful for working through trauma-related thoughts and beliefs to recontextualize traumatic memories, it is important to recognize that some traumatized individuals may not yet be able to articulate these beliefs due to the brain–body disconnect that occurs after trauma, where a lack of embodiment makes it difficult to understand or identify trauma-related thoughts (Lux et al., 2021; Shapiro, 2014; Wilson, 2002).

Similarly, while exposure therapy (Foa & Rothbaum, 1998; Rothbaum & Schwartz, 2002) targets more primal responses in the survival brain section through gradual exposure to memories and situations related to the trauma in a safe and controlled environment to promote emotional processing, it focuses on a specific memory using a top-down approach as opposed to free association of bodily traumatic responses that is observed in bottom-up approaches.

Many mindfulness-based stress reduction techniques have been incorporated into cognitive-behavioral strategies, which can help individuals to become more present and aware of their thoughts, emotions, and bodily sensations to help promote emotion regulation and dampen reactivity to traumatic reminders (Fosha, 2021; Kabat-Zinn, 2003; Segal, Williams, & Teasdale, 2018; Siegel, 2010). They can also help with training the body to be present enough to recognize automatic negative thought patterns associated with trauma as a cue to employ strategies that can help reframe negative thoughts. Dialectical behavior therapy (Linehan, 1993, 2014; Steil, Dyer, Priebe, Kleindienst, & Bohus, 2011) is another example of combining mindfulness with cognitive-behavioral techniques, where they aid in improving emotion regulation, tolerating distress, and promoting radical acceptance of a past trauma and related suffering. This encourages an individual to make a conscious effort to acknowledge and accept the pain that comes with trauma-related suffering instead of ignoring, avoiding, or wishing the situation was different, emphasizing that moving through a difficult experience allows a higher level of meaning. Often, the suppression of emotional pain associated with a lack of acceptance of trauma-related suffering requires an exhaustive amount of an individual's energy and poses a major barrier for utilizing the same energy reserve toward healing. Dialectical behavior therapy encourages an individual to be accepting of their emotional pain and reallocate that energy toward the restoration of the self. One of the earliest psychotherapeutic modalities that uses top-down principles is psychodynamic psychotherapy (Eppel, 2018; Fosha, 2002, 2021; Freud, 1896), which explores unconscious processes and primitive defense mechanisms in the context of early life experiences. This therapy is meant to help individuals explore the impact of trauma on their personality structure by identifying surface-level emotions and exploring their deeper meaning, noticing how unconscious processes create defensive mechanisms that are designed to protect the self from unpleasant or threatening thoughts and emotions. It integrates the exploration of past experiences with a focus on current issues and relationships as means to enhance insight and self-understanding. By bringing unconscious processes into awareness, individuals can gain a deeper understanding of the root causes of their difficulties and make meaningful changes.

Another necessary point of emphasis for all psychotherapeutic modalities is the power of psychoeducation in trauma, where clients are taught about how trauma can affect their thoughts, feelings, behaviors, and sensory perceptions. This can be targeted through conversations that evoke a sense of curiosity within a therapeutic community. One such example is Finding Solid Ground, a structured psychoeducational approach targeting the treatment of patients with dissociative disorders (TOPDD; Brand et al., 2022). Over the years, the work of TOPDD has brought together an international community of therapists and their clients to foster a sense of belonging through working and learning together about complex trauma and dissociative reactions that are often neglected in mainstream treatments (Brand et al., 2012, 2019; Myrick et al., 2017).

While top-down trauma treatment approaches can aid with improving higher-order functions in the prefrontal cortex, such as contextualization and reframing negative thoughts, as well as using a structured and goal-oriented approach, it requires a sturdy mind–body connection to make meaningful change. With a central focus on top-down approaches, the somatic aspects of trauma might be underemphasized, potentially leaving some individuals without a comprehensive understanding of the physical trauma response that can be all consuming. Moreover, top-down approaches primarily rely on verbal communication. This may be challenging for individuals who have difficulty expressing their emotions verbally or those who have limited access to their verbal capacities due to the nature of their trauma or symptoms of disembodiment, such as alexithymia, emotional numbing, or dissociation. Taken together, the diversity of individual responses to trauma suggests that a tailored and integrative approach may be necessary for optimal outcomes.

No One Size Fits All: Weaving the Threads of Top-Down and Bottom-Up Interventions for Trauma Treatment

In itself, there is no recipe for trauma treatment, just ingredients that can be combined in different ways as part of an integrative individualized approach. Although the traditional debate stemming from Descartes and Spinoza about dualism still emerges in treatment as therapists strive to adhere to top-down or bottom-up interventions, shifting the focus of this debate toward learning from neuroscientific evidence that demonstrates involvement of the whole brain in trauma may be the key for unifying views as both directions are necessary for trauma integration. The bottom-up general goal of being able to perceive sensations as safe may not be possible if the top-down harnessing of language and putting words to sensations is not accessible. Evidence-based trauma treatments are part of both worlds. Hence, the debate should not be on which one is a better framework but instead on how we can best help clients to process traumatic events in a neuroscientifically informed individualized way (see Bridging to Practice 9 for additional guidance).

The Collective Nature of Trauma: How Community Is Critical for Healing after Trauma

Trauma, whether experienced individually or collectively, leaves an indelible mark on communities and societies. Modern Western approaches to trauma treatment often emphasize individual healing, overlooking the profound impact of social and cultural factors. Traditional trauma treatment approaches rooted in individualism may fall short in addressing the complexities of collective trauma. By focusing solely on the individual, these approaches overlook the sociocultural context in which trauma occurs and neglect the crucial role of community support and solidarity in the healing process (Herman, 2023). Moreover, individualistic interventions may inadvertently perpetuate feelings of isolation and disconnection, further exacerbating the trauma experienced by marginalized communities.

Collectivism, in contrast to individualism, emphasizes the interconnectedness of individuals within a community or society. In collectivist cultures, such as many Indigenous communities and Eastern societies, the well-being of the group takes precedence over individual needs and desires. Here, the trauma of one member is felt by the entire group, creating a shared sense of suffering and loss. Healing from trauma becomes inherently collective, involving the participation of the entire community. Rituals, ceremonies, and traditions serve as vehicles for collective mourning, remembrance, and renewal. Similarly, in Eastern philosophies, such as Buddhism or Hinduism, the concept of interdependence underscores the interconnectedness of all beings, emphasizing compassion and empathy as central to healing. By recognizing the importance of the collective and the profound impact of sociocultural factors on trauma, trauma can be approached in a communal way that reduces the burden of loneliness, and, in turn, can expedite neuroplasticity. Here, fostering community support provides ample opportunity for individuals to trust in social bonds built with others and find solidarity, strength, and resilience in their shared experiences. In embracing collectivism, we honor the inherent dignity and interconnectedness of all beings, forging pathways toward healing, reconciliation, and collective well-being. The personal healing journey written by

Patricia Vickers below eloquently illustrates the central role of the Indigenous community in the transformation after trauma.

CASE EXAMPLE: Sm'algyax Speaking Peoples

By Patricia Vickers

Among the Gitxsan "up" the Skeena River, the Nisga'a on the Nass River and the Tsm'syen along the western Skeena River to the coast are three distinct First Nations peoples who share three dialects of the same language of Sm'algyax. I am from the village of Gitxaala on Dolphin Island where my father's mother, Kathleen Collinson, is from and where my British mother after marrying my father, was adopted into the Eagle Clan. My paternal grandfather is from the Heiltsuk community of Bella Bella and he spoke Heiltsuk, Sm'algyax, the trading language of Chinook and English. My mothers' parents immigrated separately to North America and met in Canada.

From my eighth year to when I was 11, my paternal grandparents would live with us during the winter months after we had moved to Victoria, British Columbia. Although I did not grow up in Gitxaala, I heard the language spoken when my grandparents were in our home, and the ocean tide rhythm of the language with its unique sounds were a part of me.

Gitxaala people believe there is good medicine and bad medicine. We believe that from bad medicine come curses and distortion. Colonization was openly and secretly the dissemination of bad medicine. Those who were impacted the most from the curse of colonization were children. The children experienced sexual, physical, emotional, mental, and spiritual torture in Indian residential schools, federal day schools, and foster care. Traumatic events cause a part of the soul to break away and to be imprisoned in the geographical location of the traumatic event. The curse of Indian residential schools has moved amongst us and through us as Indigenous people and is evident in our relationships with each other today. The reenactment of trauma in our close relationships is evidence of the curse and soul loss and is also known as intergenerational trauma.

The curse has changed our collective brain and distorted our consciousness through conditioning us to dehumanization.

Consciousness and Soul Loss

I was born into the curse of Indian residential schools and incest. My father was diagnosed as an incurable pedophile after my then 7-year-old daughter disclosed to me that he had been sexually abusing her and that she could not remember when it started. Her courageous disclosure precipitated in me 27 years of seeking freedom through facing dissociative amnesia, loss, grief, the source of rage and hatred, distortion of time, thought, body, and emotion—a journey of soul retrieval.

Soul Retrieval and Neurofeedback

Although not the traditional way of Gitxaala people, I adopted the sweat lodge and fasting lodge ceremonies. Under the guidance of Jack Lacerte and my eldest brother Roy, over a period of 15 years, the mystery and profound spiritual experiences of the supernatural in these ceremonies were the stable and solid foundation for 3 years of neurofeedback therapy.

In 2006, one of my family members had given me information regarding the sexual assaults throughout my childhood from 8 years of age to 13 years of age. Prior to 8 was sexual abuse from my father. After my nervous system collapsed in 2011, I was told by one of my somatic experiencing instructors that the collapse of my nervous system was due to trauma in my childhood and that a second collapse could possibly be irreparably damaging. In 2017, as clinical director of mental health and wellness with First Nations Health Authority, I took a leave of absence and contacted two colleagues asking them what I could do for the dissociative amnesia. Both colleagues, Ulrich Lanius and Steve Milstein, had spent decades working with Indigenous clients, and they introduced me to the low energy neurofeedback system. They were confident that regular sessions would assist with releasing incest memories to my mind and help with healing. Following each weekly session either the day of the session or the day after the session, I would paint a small study of the memory released to my mind that had been stored since childhood. I moved from shock, to grief, to acceptance. Step by step, session by session, I was retrieving parts of myself from the bed, basement, bedroom floor, closet, garage, and bushes at the base of a church. Slowly, ceremony from the sweat lodge and fasting lodge that taught me how to sit and sing to the darkness were teaching me to receive and welcome home the facts of my childhood. It was a digging through the layers of a life hidden, searching through my life to find my history.

Finding Home

Today, I understand that my father and mother were both conditioned to their way of being in the world. My consciousness was shaped by the curse of incest. Through neurofeedback, DBR, and traditional ceremony, I have come to understand and accept the atrocities of my childhood reality. Being with self in a compassionate, kind way is loving and nurturing self. The old way of thinking may be considered a victim's way of thinking. The ability to differentiate between a way of thinking that has the mind imprisoned to shame, guilt, and worthlessness and the present mind of a willingness to be aware, understand, and forgive are two different and separate ways and yet both are a part of my conscious living. The imprisoned or victim mind has a residue and hooks me further into powerlessness and shame—this is the mind rooted in bad medicine. The mind that is willing to understand and connect is the mind rooted in good medicine.

My eldest brother was in town and immediately my thoughts went to how he has only come to my home spontaneously a few times, and if I wanted to see him, I had to go to him. I had a sense of heaviness, a shadow over me with these thoughts. Then it all shifted when I claimed to myself that I wanted to spend time with him, and I could offer to drive him to wherever he wanted to go. He responded with childlike happiness. I provided the transportation, and we went to see boats. Because I was willing to see and understand, and our father was a fisherman, I went to learn about boats and my brother and the passion of a long line of fishermen. My relationship with my brother is different now. I am able to differentiate between thought rooted in the past and thought rooted in the present.

Neuroscience has connected me to a community of humans who understand that trauma changes the brain, that cultural oppression changes the collective brain. There is an understanding of the nature of social conditioning and distortion through shame. And neuroscience has taught me that because of the mystery and reality of neuroplasticity, the brain can heal. It is good medicine to be a part of a community that understands that dehumanization impacts all of self, that soul loss and soul retrieval and ancestral law are all vital aspects of understanding the need for healing. And above all, I'm deeply grateful for ancestral law—our songs, dances, cleansing ways, language, and ways of being—that are a part of my genetic makeup and help me walk the pathway of home.

Harnessing Neuroplasticity: A Beacon of Hope after Trauma

"I now know it's not me, it's my brain." This was a profound quote uttered by a trauma survivor upon viewing magnetic resonance imaging (MRI) images of the traumatized brain after participating in a research study. It was apparent that this epiphany was startling for the individual, as it helped to alleviate the shame that is often felt in the aftermath of trauma. Its aftermath often leaves a person feeling shattered, lost, and hopeless. However, within the realms of neuroscience lies a glimmer of optimism: neuroplasticity. Modern neuroscience has debunked the myth that the brain's development ceased in adulthood, revealing the brain's remarkable ability to change and rewire in response to our surroundings. This remarkable ability of the brain to rewire and adapt offers a beacon of hope for those navigating the arduous journey of trauma recovery. The manifestation of trauma symptoms observed in an individual is a direct result of how the brain has adapted in response to experiencing the horror and sometimes inescapable threat of trauma. However, the brain also holds the blueprint for healing, as the brain shows incredible malleability in response to the introduction of new experiences and environmental influences. This can include introducing an individual to the experience of safety, fostering the exploration of sensations in a new environment where threat is not imminent. With continued exploration at a pace that is safe to the individual, the brain can rewire to trust these safe new sensations, which evokes an individual's playful curiosity and allows for the eventual embrace of positive emotions, such as joy, love, and triumph.

By engaging in activities that stimulate the growth of new neurons and synaptic plasticity, such as movement, forming social bonds, and connecting to nature, individuals can foster the growth of new neural connections and pathways, circumventing the damage wrought by trauma. Social support plays a pivotal role in leveraging neuroplasticity for trauma recovery. Connection with others fosters a sense of safety and belonging and allows for an individual to reciprocate that same care back to the individual, activating neural circuits associated with trust and attachment. Moreover, group therapy settings also provide opportunities for individuals to share their experiences, gain validation, and receive feedback, promoting changes in neuroplasticity through interpersonal connection and support. Various therapeutic modalities leverage neuroplasticity to aid in posttrauma recovery. For example, sensorimotor intervention can promote neuroplasticity by strengthening attentional control and evoking an individual's sense of agency. By contrast, cognitive processing therapy helps individuals reframe negative thought patterns and develop coping strategies to manage trauma-related symptoms. Furthermore, DBR and EMDR allow for reprocessing traumatic memories, facilitating their integration into adaptive neural networks.

It is critical to emphasize that research is always evolving about the brain, through the introduction of new technology and the incredible strides made in modern neuroscience to study neuroplasticity—thus, we are always updating our knowledge about the body's most complex organ. While the depths of neuroscience have yet to be unveiled, it is important that we learn to trust in the brain's capacity to rebuild itself through employment of many of the vast array of treatment approaches available—no one size or approach fits all. By harnessing the brain's innate capacity to adapt and rewire, trauma survivors can cultivate resilience, reclaim agency, and forge a path where hope provides the central foundation for existence moving forward.

Hope

As a trauma survivor eloquently describes:

"What I have learned about hope is that it is not static and, at times, it can be a quest to find it. Although I probably started doubting hope from an early age, I first began to question its existence and use at the age of 20.

"Much like my journey with complex PTSD and dissociation, my journey with hope has been filled with ups and downs, belief and disbelief. When I first recognized I needed help, I was hopeful that someone could provide me with some guidance. Then, I was admitted to the hospital and my clothes were taken from me in exchange for hospital pajamas. Almost immediately, I thought something must be really wrong with me. Though I had been questioning it prior to hospitalization, I was more certain now. Next came the medications, and hope was further diminished. The fight for hope had begun.

"As I started to feel better, hope rose again and I tried to return to my life. I reached some important goals and felt hopeful about my future. Then, life turned again. It became a series of lengthy hospitalizations, increased medications, and no meaningful support. For nearly 13 years, I was living in hospitals with brief periods of respite. There were numerous diagnoses, tons of medications, and a lot of derogatory comments from health care professionals. They included but were not limited to 'only really crazy people do that' and 'frequent flyer,' which only added to my already nonexistent sense of self-worth. I also began to question my need to exist. Hope had become a deception, a lie. Who could have hope living in a hospital, doing the 'psych shuffle,' while also completely absent from the outside world?

"Numerous suicide attempts were a part of this journey. If there was hope or light, it was well buried in the deepest recesses of my mind. As far as I was concerned, hope was useless and nonexistent. Hope to me was like an abstract painting or concept. Something you try to find meaning in and can't, so you just give up on it.

"After nearly 13 years, I found myself in a small, bare room in an emergency department. I sat on the floor in a corner, knees drawn up and arms tightly wrapped around them. There were no tears, as the time for this was gone. Effectively, I might as well have been dead because this was how it felt on the inside. Then, unrecognized and unknown at the time, hope personified walked through the door that later turned out to be my therapist for the next two decades. Believe me, she was different, unlike anyone and anything I had previously encountered. She seemed gentle and kind yet turned out to be a tiger (gentle though she was).

"Little did I know then that my life or lack thereof was about to be turned upside down. She began to use curious and foreign terms to me. She talked about 'recovery.' Not that she thought something was intrinsically wrong with me but that I had experienced some really horrible things in my life. These things changed my beliefs on almost everything. I learned that these beliefs had allowed me to survive as a child but were creating chaos in my life as an adult.

"She talked about 'healing' being possible and when I challenged her, she said that there was hope and she believed in me. I said, 'There is no hope so you will need to hold it for me.' I didn't have hope and doubted I would ever have it again. There had been too many times hope had let me down. However, she agreed to hold the hope for me.

"Things didn't improve overnight. This would take time, effort, and fights. At times, I needed to be dragged kicking and screaming, much like a toddler having a tantrum. There were times I didn't like this hope that had so nonchalantly walked into my life. Sometimes, she and her team of merry helpers made me so angry, not that I'd admit that though. Anger hurt people and that was something I definitely would have no part of. Like hope, anger didn't exist for me.

"What I knew was that we were fighting for my life, though I didn't always recognize that. The small idea of fighting started to whisper inside of me. Though the whisper was nearly inaudible, it was there. Though this was a different path and would require courage, I knew there was someone willing to fight with me.

"*Stubborn* is a word that could be used to describe me and this team of helpers that included their leader. My stubbornness had met its match. This team was my match. Consistency became a part of my life, and this wasn't something that I could say had previously existed for me.

"At some point, after about 8–10 years, I announced that I was ready to take that hope back and hold it for myself again. Hope didn't return with a big flashing sign, it slowly inched back in. I haven't had to return it and hope to never have to again.

"This doesn't mean that life is without challenges or curve balls. These still and will always exist as they do for all people. As I previously stated, hope is not static, it is like the tides or 'waves on the water'; it comes in and then ebbs back. There are times when life is full of light and times when the light dims. When hope is so deeply hidden and seems nonexistent, let someone you trust hold it for some time. Just knowing someone else has it can be enough.

"I don't know if hope for me was ever truly gone. It is not a question I can really answer. What I do know is that I have found it again. I now hold it for myself. Even the smallest sliver of hope, much like the crescent moon, brings light and this sliver of light can be enough to carry you through.

"If someone you know ever asks you to hold hope for them, treat this as a gift as it has not been given lightly. You have been found so deserving and trustworthy that someone has believed that you can hold it. When they are ready to return it, be thankful for the opportunity. The person who asked you to hold it has deemed you as a gift even though they may not realize it at the time.

"Once you have given hope to someone and had it returned, be mindful that someday you too could be asked to hold and share hope for someone else. I hope that if ever someone in my life needs it, they feel I am trustworthy and ask me to hold it for them. I would consider it a great honor. Hope is a gift and the most brilliant thing about it is that it can be shared and passed from one person to another. It is not still; it has movement."

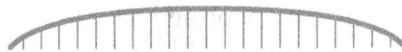

BRIDGING TO PRACTICE 9
Being with, Instead of Fixing

As integrative practitioners, our work is to find the fulcrum, balancing bottom-up and top-down strategies. This fulcrum shifts with each individual: While one requires more bottom-up sensory exploration and experiencing to reconnect to their sensations, another may need greater top-down awareness to help contextualize their intense bodily responses. In children, there is an innate drive to engage in bottom-up sensory experiencing, and the therapist (and caregiver) can incorporate top-down awareness spontaneously. When engaged in fun sensorimotor play that feels good, use of cognitive strategies (e.g., arousal charts, emotion wheels) are more fully engaged in and more readily accepted. With adults, the story may be much of the same. To fully engage with top-down strategies, their effects on arousal, affect, and bodily sensations may first need to be felt and recognized in the body to be accepted and "brought home." This approach may sound like a delicate balancing act, but it becomes a fluid dance with more experience and advanced professional reasoning. This integrative approach also requires a great deal of open-mindedness on the part of the therapist and a relinquishing of control in service of the client's shifting needs over time.

As therapists, we must have the modesty to accept that no level of professional training or learned techniques are above the inner wisdom of the client. It is our job not to fix but to foster the therapeutic holding space to invite this wisdom to come to the surface. Much of the work here is on the part of the therapist: relinquishing control and the need to talk, do, or otherwise prove to our clients (and ourselves) that we are "doing something." As we have discussed in this book, there is much more than meets the eye with bottom-up treatments that act on preverbal levels of the survival brain. We must sometimes learn to be silent and tap into our own bodily state in order to be fully attuned and open to our client's full experience.

In order for our clients to sense our attuned presence, we must be grounded and regulated ourselves. This is difficult work, perhaps the most difficult work we can encounter as mental health professionals. Understanding our own self-regulation needs and responses (triggers) to our clients is paramount and prerequisite for holding space and fully attuning to another. Therapists must invest just as much time attending to their own regulatory needs and fostering attachment to inner bodily experience as they do when they attempt to heal others.

Questions therapists can ask themselves:

1. What moments do I feel most connected or attuned to my client? Where do I feel that in my body?
2. When do I feel unattuned or confused as to how my client is feeling? Where do I feel that in my body?
3. What do I do to regulate myself before or after a difficult day? What sensory input does this activity inherently involve?

References

Addis, D. R., Moscovitch, M., Crawley, A. P., & McAndrews, M. P. (2004). Recollective qualities modulate hippocampal activation during autobiographical memory retrieval. *Hippocampus, 14*(6), 752–762.

Addy, P. H., Garcia-Romeu, A., Metzger, M., & Wade, J. (2015). The subjective experience of acute, experimentally-induced *Salvia divinorum* inebriation. *Journal of Psychopharmacology, 29*(4), 426–435.

Adler, G. K., & Geenen, R. (2005). Hypothalamic–pituitary–adrenal and autonomic nervous system functioning in fibromyalgia. *Rheumatic Disease Clinics, 31*(1), 187–202.

Adolphs, R. (2002). Neural systems for recognizing emotion. *Current Opinion in Neurobiology, 12*(2), 169–177.

Ahn, S. K., & Balaban, C. D. (2010). Distribution of 5-HT1B and 5-HT1D receptors in the inner ear. *Brain Research, 1346*, 92–101.

Ainsworth, M. D. S. (1978). The Bowlby–Ainsworth attachment theory. *Behavioral and Brain Sciences, 1*(3), 436–438.

Akbarian, S., Berndl, K., Grusser, O. J., Guldin, W., Pause, M., & Schreiter, U. (1988). Responses of single neurons in the parietoinsular vestibular cortex of primates. *Annals of the New York Academy of Sciences, 545*, 187–202.

Akiki, T. J., Averill, C. L., Wrocklage, K. M., Scott, J. C., Averill, L. A., Schweinsburg, B., et al. (2018). Default mode network abnormalities in posttraumatic stress disorder: A novel network-restricted topology approach. *NeuroImage, 176*, 489–498.

Alboni, P., & Alboni, M. (2014). Vasovagal syncope as a manifestation of an evolutionary selected trait. *Journal of Atrial Fibrillation, 7*(2), 1035.

Alcaro, A., & Panksepp, J. (2011). The SEEKING mind: Primal neuro-affective substrates for appetitive incentive states and their pathological dynamics in addictions and depression. *Neuroscience and Biobehavioral Reviews, 35*(9), 1805–1820.

Alm, P. A. (2004). Stuttering, emotions, and heart rate during anticipatory anxiety: A critical review. *Journal of Fluency Disorders, 29*(2), 123–133.

Anastasopoulos, D., Naushahi, J., Sklavos, S., & Bronstein, A. M. (2015). Fast gaze reorientations by combined movements of the eye, head, trunk and lower extremities. *Experimental Brain Research, 233*(5), 1639–1650.

Angelopoulou, E., & Drigas, A. (2021). Working memory, attention and their relationship: A theoretical overview. *Research, Society and Development, 10*(5), e46410515288.

Anzellotti, S., & Caramazza, A. (2017). Multimodal representations of person identity individuated with fMRI. *Cortex, 89,* 85–97.

Asmundson, G. J., Norton, G. R., Allerdings, M. D., Norton, P. J., & Larsen, D. K. (1998). Posttraumatic stress disorder and work-related injury. *Journal of Anxiety Disorders, 12*(1), 57–69.

Ayres, A. J. (1972). *Sensory integration and learning disorders.* Western Psychological Services.

Ayres, A. J., & Robbins, J. (2005). *Sensory integration and the child: Understanding hidden sensory challenges.* Western Psychological Services.

Baddeley, A., Lewis, V., Eldridge, M., & Thomson, N. (1984). Attention and retrieval from long-term memory. *Journal of Experimental Psychology: General, 113*(4), 518–540.

Baier, B., zu Eulenburg, P., Best, C., Geber, C., Muller-Forell, W., Birklein, F., et al. (2013). Posterior insular cortex—A site of vestibular–somatosensory interaction? *Brain and Behavior, 3*(5), 519–524.

Bak, M., Girvin, J. P., Hambrecht, F. T., Kufta, C. V., Loeb, G. E., & Schmidt, E. M. (1990). Visual sensations produced by intracortical microstimulation of the human occipital cortex. *Medical and Biological Engineering and Computing, 28*(3), 257–259.

Bandler, R., Keay, K. A., Floyd, N., & Price, J. (2000). Central circuits mediating patterned autonomic activity during active vs. passive emotional coping. *Brain Research Bulletin, 53*(1), 95–104.

Barrett, L. F. (2017). *How emotions are made: The secret life of the brain.* Houghton Mifflin Harcourt.

Bassett, D. S., & Gazzaniga, M. S. (2011). Understanding complexity in the human brain. *Trends in Cognitive Sciences, 15*(5), 200–209.

Beck, J. S. (2021). *Cognitive behavior therapy: Basics and beyond* (3rd ed.). Guilford Press.

Beiser, D. G., & Houk, J. C. (1998). Model of cortical–basal ganglionic processing: Encoding the serial order of sensory events. *Journal of Neurophysiology, 79*(6), 3168–3188.

Bell, A. G. (1880). On the production and reproduction of sound by light. *American Journal of Science, s3-20*(118), 305–324.

Bentham, J. (1780). *An introduction to the principles of morals and legislation* (Vol. 45). Dover.

Berardi, N., Pizzorusso, T., & Maffei, L. (2000). Critical periods during sensory development. *Current Opinion in Neurobiology, 10*(1), 138–145.

Bergmann, U. (2008). The neurobiology of EMDR: Exploring the thalamus and neural integration. *Journal of EMDR Practice and Research, 2*(4), 300–314.

Bergouignan, L., Nyberg, L., & Ehrsson, H. H. (2014). Out-of-body-induced hippocampal amnesia. *Proceedings of the National Academy of Sciences of the United States of America, 111*(12), 4421–4426.

Bergouignan, L., Nyberg, L., & Ehrsson, H. H. (2022). Out-of-body memory encoding causes third-person perspective at recall. *Journal of Cognitive Psychology, 34*(1), 160–178.

Berntson, G. G., & Khalsa, S. S. (2021). Neural circuits of interoception. *Trends in Neuroscience, 44*(1), 17–28.

Berthoud, H. R., & Neuhuber, W. L. (2000). Functional and chemical anatomy of the afferent vagal system. *Autonomic Neuroscience: Basic and Clinical, 85*(1–3), 1–17.

Best, C., Eckhardt-Henn, A., Diener, G., Bense, S., Breuer, P., & Dieterich, M. (2006). Interaction of somatoform and vestibular disorders. *Journal of Neurology, Neurosurgery, and Psychiatry, 77*(5), 658–664.

Blanke, O., & Arzy, S. (2005). The out-of-body experience: Disturbed self-processing at the temporo–parietal junction. *Neuroscientist, 11*(1), 16–24.

Bluhm, R. L., Williamson, P. C., Osuch, E. A., Frewen, P. A., Stevens, T. K., Boksman, K., et al. (2009). Alterations in default network connectivity in posttraumatic stress disorder related to early-life trauma. *Journal of Psychiatry and Neuroscience, 34*(3), 187–194.

Bolmont, B., Gangloff, P., Vouriot, A., & Perrin, P. P. (2002). Mood states and anxiety influence abilities to maintain balance control in healthy human subjects. *Neuroscience Letters, 329*(1), 96–100.

Bornstein, M. H., & Esposito, G. (2023). Coregulation: A multilevel approach via biology and behavior. *Children, 10*(8), 1323.

Bowlby, J. (1979). The Bowlby–Ainsworth attachment theory. *Behavioral and Brain Sciences, 2*(4), 637–638.

Brand, B., McNary, S., Myrick, A., Classen, C., Lanius, R., Loewenstein, R., et al. (2012). A longitudinal naturalistic study of patients with dissociative disorders treated by community clinicians. *Psychological Trauma: Theory Research Practice and Policy, 5*, 301–308.

Brand, B. L., Schielke, H. J., Putnam, K. T., Putnam, F. W., Loewenstein, R. J., Myrick, A., et al. (2019). An online educational program for individuals with dissociative disorders and their clinicians: 1-year and 2-year follow-up. *Journal of Traumatic Stress, 32*(1), 156–166.

Brand, B. L., Schielke, H., Schiavone, F., & Lanius, R. A. (2022). *Finding solid ground: Overcoming obstacles in trauma treatment*. Oxford University Press.

Breit, S., Kupferberg, A., Rogler, G., & Hasler, G. (2018). Vagus nerve as modulator of the brain–gut axis in psychiatric and inflammatory disorders. *Frontiers in Psychiatry, 9*, 44.

Bretherton, I. (1992). The origins of attachment theory: John Bowlby and Mary Ainsworth. *Developmental Psychology, 28*(5), 759–775.

Brewin, C. R. (2014). Episodic memory, perceptual memory, and their interaction: Foundations for a theory of posttraumatic stress disorder. *Psychological Bulletin, 140*(1), 69–97.

Brewin, C. R., Dalgleish, T., & Joseph, S. (1996). A dual representation theory of posttraumatic stress disorder. *Psychological Review, 103*(4), 670–686.

Briere, J. (1988). The long-term clinical correlates of childhood sexual victimization. *Annals of the New York Academy of Sciences, 528*, 327–334.

Briere, J. N. (1992). *Child abuse trauma: Theory and treatment of the lasting effects*. Sage.

Briere, J. (2019). *Treating risky and compulsive behavior in trauma survivors*. Guilford Press.

Briere, J., & Elliott, D. M. (2003). Prevalence and psychological sequelae of self-reported childhood physical and sexual abuse in a general population sample of men and women. *Child Abuse and Neglect, 27*(10), 1205–1222.

Briere, J., Hodges, M., & Godbout, N. (2010). Traumatic stress, affect dysregulation, and dysfunctional avoidance: A structural equation model. *Journal of Traumatic Stress, 23*(6), 767–774.

Briere, J., Kaltman, S., & Green, B. L. (2008). Accumulated childhood trauma and symptom complexity. *Journal of Traumatic Stress, 21*(2), 223–226.

Briere, J. N., & Lanktree, C. B. (2011). *Treating complex trauma in adolescents and young adults*. Sage.

Briere, J., & Runtz, M. (1990). Differential adult symptomatology associated with three types of child abuse histories. *Child Abuse and Neglect, 14*(3), 357–364.

Briere, J., Runtz, M., & Rodd, K. (2024). Child and adolescent exposure to sexual harassment: Relationship to gender, contact sexual abuse, and adult psychological symptoms. *Journal of Interpersonal Violence, 39*(13–14), 2981–2996.

Brom, D., Stokar, Y., Lawi, C., Nuriel-Porat, V., Ziv, Y., Lerner, K., et al. (2017). Somatic experiencing for posttraumatic stress disorder: A randomized controlled outcome study. *Journal of Traumatic Stress, 30*(3), 304–312.

Brown, A., Tse, T., & Fortune, T. (2019). Defining sensory modulation: A review of the concept and a contemporary definition for application by occupational therapists. *Scandinavian Journal of Occupational Therapy, 26*(7), 515–523.

Brown, H., Adams, R. A., Parees, I., Edwards, M., & Friston, K. (2013). Active inference, sensory attenuation and illusions. *Cognitive Processing, 14*(4), 411–427.

Bryant-Davis, T. (2007). Healing requires recognition: The case for race-based traumatic stress. *The Counseling Psychologist, 35*(1), 135–143.

Bryant-Davis, T., Chung, H., & Tillman, S. (2009). From the margins to the center: Ethnic minority women and the mental health effects of sexual assault. *Trauma, Violence, and Abuse, 10*(4), 330–357.

Buckner, R. L., Andrews-Hanna, J. R., & Schacter, D. L. (2008). The brain's default network: Anatomy, function, and relevance to disease. *Annals of the New York Academy of Sciences, 1124*, 1–38.

Burgess, N., & Hitch, G. J. (2006). A revised model of short-term memory and long-term learning of verbal sequences. *Journal of Memory and Language, 55*(4), 627–652.

Butler, E. A., & Randall, A. K. (2013). Emotional coregulation in close relationships. *Emotion Review, 5*(2), 202–210.

Byron, B., & Alfredo, A. (2016). From hearing sounds to recognizing phonemes: Primary auditory cortex is a truly perceptual language area. *AIMS Neuroscience, 3*(4), 454–473.

Cabeza, R., & St Jacques, P. (2007). Functional neuroimaging of autobiographical memory. *Trends in Cognitive Sciences, 11*(5), 219–227.

Calder, A. J., Keane, J., Manes, F., Antoun, N., & Young, A. W. (2000). Impaired recognition and experience of disgust following brain injury. *Nature Neuroscience, 3*(11), 1077–1078.

Carhart-Harris, R. L., Leech, R., Hellyer, P. J., Shanahan, M., Feilding, A., Tagliazucchi, E., et al. (2014). The entropic brain: A theory of conscious states informed by neuroimaging research with psychedelic drugs. *Frontiers in Human Neuroscience, 8*, 55875.

Cassilhas, R. C., Tufik, S., & de Mello, M. T. (2016). Physical exercise, neuroplasticity, spatial learning and memory. *Cellular and Molecular Life Sciences, 73*(5), 975–983.

Catani, M., Dell'acqua, F., & Thiebaut de Schotten, M. (2013). A revised limbic system model for memory, emotion and behaviour. *Neuroscience and Biobehavioral Reviews, 37*(8), 1724–1737.

Cauzzo, S., Singh, K., Stauder, M., Garcia-Gomar, M. G., Vanello, N., Passino, C., et al. (2022). Functional connectome of brainstem nuclei involved in autonomic, limbic, pain and sensory processing in living humans from 7 Tesla resting state fMRI. *NeuroImage, 250*, 118925.

Champagne, T. (2011). The influence of posttraumatic stress disorder, depression, and sensory processing patterns on occupational engagement: A case study. *Work, 38*(1), 67–75.

Chapman, H. A., Kim, D. A., Susskind, J. M., & Anderson, A. K. (2009). In bad taste: Evidence for the oral origins of moral disgust. *Science, 323*, 1222–1226.

Chaposhloo, M., Nicholson, A. A., Becker, S., McKinnon, M. C., Lanius, R., & Shaw, S. B. (2023). Altered resting-state functional connectivity in the anterior and posterior hippocampus in post-traumatic stress disorder: The central role of the anterior hippocampus. *NeuroImage: Clinical, 38*, 103417.

Chen, A. C., & Etkin, A. (2013). Hippocampal network connectivity and activation differentiates post-traumatic stress disorder from generalized anxiety disorder. *Neuropsychopharmacology, 38*(10), 1889–1898.

Chen, R., Yaseen, Z., Cohen, L. G., & Hallett, M. (1998). Time course of corticospinal excitability in reaction time and self-paced movements. *Annals of Neurology, 44*(3), 317–325.

Chesterton, G. K. (1905). *Heretics* (12th ed.). John Lane.

Ciaunica, A., Safron, A., & Delafield-Butt, J. (2021). Back to square one: The bodily roots of conscious experiences in early life. *Neuroscience of Consciousness, 2021*(2), niab037.

Clancy, K. J., Devignes, Q., Ren, B., Pollmann, Y., Nielsen, S. R., Howell, K., et al. (2024). Spatiotemporal dynamics of hippocampal–cortical networks underlying the unique phenomenological properties of trauma-related intrusive memories. *Molecular Psychiatry, 29*, 2161–2169.

Classen, C. C., Hughes, L., Clark, C., Hill Mohammed, B., Woods, P., & Beckett, B. (2021). A pilot RCT of a body-oriented group therapy for complex trauma survivors: An adaptation of sensorimotor psychotherapy. *Journal of Trauma and Dissociation, 22*(1), 52–68.

Coan, J. A., Schaefer, H. S., & Davidson, R. J. (2006). Lending a hand: Social regulation of the neural response to threat. *Psychological Science, 17*(12), 1032–1039.

Cohen, J. (1980). Structural consequences of psychic trauma: A new look at "Beyond the Pleasure Principle." *International Journal of Psychoanalysis, 61*(3), 421–432.

Cohn, R. (2021). *Working with the developmental trauma of childhood neglect: Using psychotherapy and attachment theory techniques in clinical practice.* Routledge.

Corneil, B. D., Munoz, D. P., Chapman, B. B., Admans, T., & Cushing, S. L. (2008). Neuromuscular consequences of reflexive covert orienting. *Nature Neuroscience, 11*(1), 13–15.

Corneil, B. D., Olivier, E., & Munoz, D. P. (2002). Neck muscle responses to stimulation of monkey superior colliculus. I. Topography and manipulation of stimulation parameters. *Journal of Neurophysiology, 88*(4), 1980–1999.

Corrigan, F. M., & Christie-Sands, J. (2020). An innate brainstem self–other system involving orienting, affective responding, and polyvalent relational seeking: Some clinical implications for a "deep brain reorienting" trauma psychotherapy approach. *Medical Hypotheses, 136,* 109502.

Corrigan, F. M., Fisher, J. J., & Nutt, D. J. (2011). Autonomic dysregulation and the window of tolerance model of the effects of complex emotional trauma. *Journal of Psychopharmacology, 25*(1), 17–25.

Corrigan, F., & Grand, D. (2013). Brainspotting: Recruiting the midbrain for accessing and healing sensorimotor memories of traumatic activation. *Medical Hypotheses, 80*(6), 759–766.

Corrigan, F. M., Young, H., & Christie-Sands, J. (2024). *Deep brain reorienting: Understanding the neuroscience of trauma, attachment wounding, and DBR psychotherapy.* Taylor & Francis.

Cox, A. D., Fesik, S. W., Kimmelman, A. C., Luo, J., & Der, C. J. (2014). Drugging the undruggable RAS: Mission possible? *Nature Reviews: Drug Discovery, 13*(11), 828–851.

Craig, A. D. (2003). Interoception: The sense of the physiological condition of the body. *Current Opinion in Neurobiology, 13*(4), 500–505.

Craig, A. D. (2009). How do you feel—now?: The anterior insula and human awareness. *Nature Reviews: Neuroscience, 10*(1), 59–70.

Cramer, G. D., & Darby, S. A. (2014). *Clinical anatomy of the spine, spinal cord, and ANS.* Elsevier.

Crenna, P., & Frigo, C. (1991). A motor programme for the initiation of forward-oriented movements in humans. *Journal of Physiology, 437*(1), 635–653.

Crick, F. H. (1979). Thinking about the brain. *Scientific American, 241*(3), 219–232.

Critchley, H. D., & Garfinkel, S. N. (2017). Interoception and emotion. *Current Opinion in Psychology, 17,* 7–14.

Croy, I., Drechsler, E., Hamilton, P., Hummel, T., & Olausson, H. (2016). Olfactory modulation of affective touch processing—A neurophysiological investigation. *NeuroImage, 135,* 135–141.

Cullen, K. E., & Chacron, M. J. (2023). Neural substrates of perception in the vestibular thalamus during natural self-motion: A review. *Current Research in Neurobiology, 4,* 100073.

Damasio, A. R. (1998). Emotion in the perspective of an integrated nervous system. *Brain Research: Brain Research Reviews, 26*(2–3), 83–86.

Damasio, A. R. (2003). *Looking for Spinoza: Joy, sorrow, and the feeling brain.* Harcourt.

Dana, D. (2018). *The polyvagal theory in therapy: Engaging the rhythm of regulation.* Norton.

d'Andrea, W., Pole, N., DePierro, J., Freed, S., & Wallace, D. B. (2013). Heterogeneity of defensive responses after exposure to trauma: Blunted autonomic reactivity in response to startling sounds. *International Journal of Psychophysiology, 90*(1), 80–89.

Daniels, J. K., McFarlane, A. C., Bluhm, R. L., Moores, K. A., Clark, C. R., Shaw, M. E., et al. (2010). Switching between executive and default mode networks in posttraumatic stress disorder: Alterations in functional connectivity. *Journal of Psychiatry and Neuroscience, 35*(4), 258–266.

Daniels, J. K., & Vermetten, E. (2016). Odor-induced recall of emotional memories in PTSD—Review and new paradigm for research. *Experimental Neurology, 284*(Pt. B), 168–180.

Davidson, R. J., & McEwen, B. S. (2012). Social influences on neuroplasticity: Stress and interventions to promote well-being. *Nature Neuroscience, 15*(5), 689–695.

Day, B. L., & Fitzpatrick, R. C. (2005). The vestibular system. *Current Biology, 15*(15), R583–586.

De Kloet, E. R. (2004). Hormones and the stressed brain. *Annals of the New York Academy of Sciences, 1018*(1), 1–15.

Dehay, C., & Kennedy, H. (2020). Evolution of the human brain. *Science, 369*, 506–507.

DeMaster, D., Pathman, T., Lee, J. K., & Ghetti, S. (2014). Structural development of the hippocampus and episodic memory: Developmental differences along the anterior/posterior axis. *Cerebral Cortex, 24*(11), 3036–3045.

Deroualle, D., Borel, L., Deveze, A., & Lopez, C. (2015). Changing perspective: The role of vestibular signals. *Neuropsychologia, 79*(Pt. B), 175–185.

Deroualle, D., & Lopez, C. (2014). Toward a vestibular contribution to social cognition. *Frontiers in Integrative Neuroscience, 8*, 16.

Derryberry, D., & Tucker, D. M. (1992). Neural mechanisms of emotion. *Journal of Consulting and Clinical Psychology, 60*(3), 329–338.

Devlin, J. T., Raley, J., Tunbridge, E., Lanary, K., Floyer-Lea, A., Narain, C., et al. (2003). Functional asymmetry for auditory processing in human primary auditory cortex. *Journal of Neuroscience, 23*(37), 11516–11522.

DeWitt, I., & Rauschecker, J. P. (2013). Wernicke's area revisited: Parallel streams and word processing. *Brain and Language, 127*(2), 181–191.

Diekelmann, S., Wilhelm, I., & Born, J. (2009). The whats and whens of sleep-dependent memory consolidation. *Sleep Medicine Reviews, 13*(5), 309–321.

Drescher, K. D., Foy, D. W., Kelly, C., Leshner, A., Schutz, K., & Litz, B. (2011). An exploration of the viability and usefulness of the construct of moral injury in war veterans. *Traumatology, 17*(1), 8–13.

Dudine, L., Canaletti, C., Giudici, F., Lunardelli, A., Abram, G., Santini, I., et al. (2021). Investigation on the loss of taste and smell and consequent psychological effects: A cross-sectional study on healthcare workers who contracted the COVID-19 infection. *Frontiers in Public Health, 9*, 666442.

Duek, O., Seidemann, R., Pietrzak, R. H., & Harpaz-Rotem, I. (2023). Distinguishing emotional numbing symptoms of posttraumatic stress disorder from major depressive disorder. *Journal of Affective Disorders, 324*, 294–299.

Dunn, W. (1997). The impact of sensory processing abilities on the daily lives of young children and their families: A conceptual model. *Infants and Young Children, 9*(4), 23–35.

Edwards, E. R. (2022). Posttraumatic stress and alexithymia: A meta-analysis of presentation and severity. *Psychological Trauma: Theory, Research, Practice, and Policy, 14*(7), 1192–1200.

Elbasheir, A., Bond, R., Harnett, N. G., Guelfo, A., Karkare, M. C., Fulton, T. M., et al. (in press). Racial discrimination-related interoceptive network disruptions: A pathway to disconnection. *Biological Psychiatry.*

Emerson, D., & Hopper, E. (2011). *Overcoming trauma through yoga: Reclaiming your body.* North Atlantic Books.

Engel-Yeger, B., Palgy-Levin, D., & Lev-Wiesel, R. (2013). The sensory profile of people with post-traumatic stress symptoms. *Occupational Therapy in Mental Health, 29*(3), 266–278.

Eppel, A. (2018). *Short-term psychodynamic psychotherapy.* Springer.

Eskine, K. J., Kacinik, N. A., & Prinz, J. J. (2011). A bad taste in the mouth: Gustatory disgust influences moral judgment. *Psychological Science, 22*(3), 295–299.

Fani, N., Carter, S. E., Harnett, N. G., Ressler, K. J., & Bradley, B. (2021). Association of racial discrimination with neural response to threat in Black women in the US exposed to trauma. *JAMA Psychiatry, 78*(9), 1005–1012.

Fani, N., Fulton, T., & Botzanowski, B. (2024). The neurophysiology of interoceptive disruptions in trauma-exposed populations. In *Current topics in behavioral neuroscience* (pp. 1–28). Springer.

Farb, N. A., Segal, Z. V., & Anderson, A. K. (2013). Mindfulness meditation training alters cortical representations of interoceptive attention. *Social Cognitive and Affective Neuroscience, 8*(1), 15–26.

Farina, B., Liotti, M., & Imperatori, C. (2019). The role of attachment trauma and disintegrative pathogenic processes in the traumatic-dissociative dimension. *Frontiers in Psychology, 10,* 933.

Farrant, K., & Uddin, L. Q. (2015). Asymmetric development of dorsal and ventral attention networks in the human brain. *Developmental Cognitive Neuroscience, 12,* 165–174.

Feldman, R. (2007). Parent–infant synchrony and the construction of shared timing; physiological precursors, developmental outcomes, and risk conditions. *Journal of Child Psychology and Psychiatry, 48*(3–4), 329–354.

Felitti, V. J., Anda, R. F., Nordenberg, D., Williamson, D. F., Spitz, A. M., Edwards, V., et al. (1998). Relationship of childhood abuse and household dysfunction to many of the leading causes of death in adults: The Adverse Childhood Experiences (ACE) study. *American Journal of Preventative Medicine, 14*(4), 245–258.

Fenster, R. J., Lebois, L. A. M., Ressler, K. J., & Suh, J. (2018). Brain circuit dysfunction in post-traumatic stress disorder: From mouse to man. *Nature Reviews: Neuroscience, 19*(9), 535–551.

Ferrè, E. R., & Haggard, P. (2015). Vestibular–somatosensory interactions: A mechanism in search of a function? *Multisensory Research, 28*(5–6), 559–579.

Ferrè, E. R., Vagnoni, E., & Haggard, P. (2013). Vestibular contributions to bodily awareness. *Neuropsychologia, 51*(8), 1445–1452.

Ferrer, E., & Helm, J. L. (2013). Dynamical systems modeling of physiological coregulation in dyadic interactions. *International Journal of Psychophysiology, 88*(3), 296–308.

Finn, H., Warner, E., Price, M., & Spinazzola, J. (2018). The boy who was hit in the face: Somatic regulation and processing of preverbal complex trauma. *Journal of Child and Adolescent Trauma, 11*(3), 277–288.

Fisher, J. (2017). *Healing the fragmented selves of trauma survivors: Overcoming internal self-alienation.* Routledge.

Fisher, J., & Ogden, P. (2009). Sensorimotor psychotherapy. In C. A. Courtois & J. D. Ford (Eds.), *Treating complex traumatic stress disorders: An evidence-based guide* (pp. 312–328). Guilford Press.

Fisher, S. F. (2014). *Neurofeedback in the treatment of developmental trauma: Calming the fear-driven brain.* Norton.

Flavell, J. H., & Miller, P. H. (1998). Social cognition. In W. Damon (Ed.), *Handbook of child psychology: Vol. 2. Cognition, perception, and language* (pp. 851–898). Wiley.

Foa, E. B., Ehlers, A., Clark, D. M., Tolin, D. F., & Orsillo, S. M. (1999). The Posttraumatic Cognitions Inventory (PTCI): Development and validation. *Psychological Assessment, 11*(3), 303–314.

Foa, E. B., & Rothbaum, B. O. (1998). *Treating the trauma of rape: Cognitive-behavioral therapy for PTSD.* Guilford Press.

Fonzo, G. A., Goodkind, M. S., Oathes, D. J., Zaiko, Y. V., Harvey, M., Peng, K. K., et al. (2017). PTSD psychotherapy outcome predicted by brain activation during emotional reactivity and regulation. *American Journal of Psychiatry, 174*(12), 1163–1174.

Fosha, D. (2001). The dyadic regulation of affect. *Journal of Clinical Psychology, 57*(2), 227–242.

Fosha, D. (2002). The activation of affective change processes in accelerated experiential-dynamic psychotherapy (AEDP). In F. W. Kaslow & J. J. Magnavita (Eds.), *Comprehensive handbook of psychotherapy: Vol. 1. Psychodynamic/object relations* (pp. 309–343). Wiley.

Fosha, D. (2005). Emotion, true self, true other, core state: Toward a clinical theory of affective change process. *Psychoanalytic Review, 92*(4), 513–551.

Fosha, D. (2013). A heaven in a wild flower: Self, dissociation, and treatment in the context of the neurobiological core self. *Psychoanalytic Inquiry, 33*(5), 496–523.

Fosha, D. (2021). *Undoing aloneness and the transformation of suffering into flourishing: AEDP 2.0.* American Psychological Association.

Frankland, P. W., Josselyn, S. A., & Kohler, S. (2019). The neurobiological foundation of memory retrieval. *Nature Neuroscience, 22*(10), 1576–1585.

Freud, S. (1896). The aetiology of hysteria. In J. Strachey (Trans.), *The standard edition of the complete psychological works of Sigmund Freud* (Vol. 3, pp. 187–221). Hogarth Press.

Frewen, P. A., Dozois, D. J. A., Neufeld, R. W. J., Lane, R. D., Densmore, M., Stevens, T. K., et al. (2010). Individual differences in trait mindfulness predict dorsomedial prefrontal and amygdala response during emotional imagery: An fMRI study. *Personality and Individual Differences, 49*(5), 479–484.

Frewen, P. A., Dozois, D. J., Neufeld, R. W., Lane, R. D., Densmore, M., Stevens, T. K., et al. (2012). Emotional numbing in posttraumatic stress disorder: A functional magnetic resonance imaging study. *Journal of Clinical Psychiatry, 73*(4), 431–436.

Frewen, P. A., Dozois, D. J., Neufeld, R. W., & Lanius, R. A. (2008). Meta-analysis of alexithymia in posttraumatic stress disorder. *Journal of Traumatic Stress, 21*(2), 243–246.

Frewen, P., Lane, R. D., Neufeld, R. W., Densmore, M., Stevens, T., & Lanius, R. (2008). Neural correlates of levels of emotional awareness during trauma script-imagery in posttraumatic stress disorder. *Psychosomatic Medicine, 70*(1), 27–31.

Frewen, P. A., & Lanius, R. A. (2006). Toward a psychobiology of posttraumatic self-dysregulation: Reexperiencing, hyperarousal, dissociation, and emotional numbing. *Annals of the New York Academy of Sciences, 1071*, 110–124.

Frewen, P., & Lanius, R. (2015). *Healing the traumatized self: Consciousness, neuroscience, treatment.* Norton.

Frewen, P. A., Lanius, R. A., Dozois, D. J., Neufeld, R. W., Pain, C., Hopper, J. W., et al. (2008). Clinical and neural correlates of alexithymia in posttraumatic stress disorder. *Journal of Abnormal Psychology, 117*(1), 171–181.

Frewen, P., Schroeter, M. L., Riva, G., Cipresso, P., Fairfield, B., Padulo, C., et al. (2020). Neuroimaging the consciousness of self: Review, and conceptual–methodological framework. *Neuroscience and Biobehavioral Reviews, 112*, 164–212.

Friston, K. (2010). The free-energy principle: A unified brain theory? *Nature Reviews: Neuroscience, 11*(2), 127–138.

Friston, K., FitzGerald, T., Rigoli, F., Schwartenbeck, P., & Pezzulo, G. (2017). Active inference: A process theory. *Neural Computation, 29*(1), 1–49.

Friston, K., Kilner, J., & Harrison, L. (2006). A free energy principle for the brain. *Journal of Physiology: Paris, 100*(1–3), 70–87.

Friston, K., Mattout, J., & Kilner, J. (2011). Action understanding and active inference. *Biological Cybernetics, 104*(1–2), 137–160.

Frith, C., & Frith, U. (2005). Theory of mind. *Current Biology, 15*(17), R644–646.

Fuller, T. (1732). *Gnomologia: Adagies and proverbs; Wise sentences and witty sayings, ancient and modern, foreign and British.* Barker.

Furman, J. M., & Marcus, D. A. (2012). Migraine and motion sensitivity. *CONTINUUM: Lifelong Learning in Neurology, 18*(5 Neuro-otology), 1102–1117.

Gallagher, M., Kearney, B., & Ferrè, E. R. (2021). Where is my hand in space?: The internal model of gravity influences proprioception. *Biology Letters, 17*(6), 20210115.

Gallup, G. G., & Rager, D. R. (1996). Tonic immobility as a model of extreme states of behavioral inhibition: Issues of methodology and measurement. In P. R. Sanberg, K. P. Ossenkopp, & M. Kavaliers (Eds.), *Motor activity and movement disorders: Contemporary neuroscience* (pp. 57–80). Humana Press.

Gattuso, J. J., Perkins, D., Ruffell, S., Lawrence, A. J., Hoyer, D., Jacobson, L. H., et al. (2023).

Default mode network modulation by psychedelics: A systematic review. *International Journal of Neuropsychopharmacology, 26*(3), 155–188.

Gene-Cos, N., Fisher, J., Ogden, P., & Cantrell, A. (2016). Sensorimotor psychotherapy group therapy in the treatment of complex PTSD. *Annals of Psychiatry and Mental Health, 4*(6), 1080.

Geuze, E., Westenberg, H. G., Jochims, A., de Kloet, C. S., Bohus, M., Vermetten, E., et al. (2007). Altered pain processing in veterans with posttraumatic stress disorder. *Archives of General Psychiatry, 64*(1), 76–85.

Giraud, M., Zapparoli, L., Basso, G., Petilli, M., Paulesu, E., & Nava, E. (2024). Mapping the emotional homunculus with fMRI. *iScience, 27*(6), 109985.

Goelet, P., Castellucci, V. F., Schacher, S., & Kandel, E. R. (1986). The long and the short of long-term memory—A molecular framework. *Nature, 322*, 419–422.

Goldberg, J. M., Wilson, V. J., Cullen, K. E., Angelaki, D. E., Broussard, D. M., Buttner-Ennever, J. F., et al. (2012). *The vestibular system: A sixth sense.* Oxford University Press.

Golkar, A., Lonsdorf, T. B., Olsson, A., Lindstrom, K. M., Berrebi, J., Fransson, P., et al. (2012). Distinct contributions of the dorsolateral prefrontal and orbitofrontal cortex during emotion regulation. *PLoS One, 7*(11), e48107.

Goodyear-Brown, P. (2009). *Play therapy with traumatized children.* Wiley.

Graf, W., & Klam, F. (2006). Le système vestibulaire: Anatomie fonctionnelle et comparée, evolution et développement. *Comptes Rendus Palevol, 5*(3–4), 637–655.

Graham, K., Searle, A., Van Hooff, M., Lawrence-Wood, E., & McFarlane, A. (2019). The associations between physical and psychological symptoms and traumatic military deployment exposures. *Journal of Traumatic Stress, 32*(6), 957–966.

Gray, P., Lancy, D. F., & Bjorklund, D. F. (2023). Decline in independent activity as a cause of decline in children's mental well-being: Summary of the evidence. *Journal of Pediatrics, 260*, 113352.

Greenberg, L. S., & Goldman, R. N. (2019). *Clinical handbook of emotion-focused therapy.* American Psychological Association.

Greicius, M. D., Krasnow, B., Reiss, A. L., & Menon, V. (2003). Functional connectivity in the resting brain: A network analysis of the default mode hypothesis. *Proceedings of the National Academy of Sciences, 100*(1), 253–258.

Halberstadt, A. L., & Balaban, C. D. (2006). Serotonergic and nonserotonergic neurons in the dorsal raphe nucleus send collateralized projections to both the vestibular nuclei and the central amygdaloid nucleus. *Neuroscience, 140*(3), 1067–1077.

Handel, S. (1993). *Listening: An introduction to the perception of auditory events.* MIT Press.

Hansel, A., & von Kanel, R. (2008). The ventro–medial prefrontal cortex: A major link between the autonomic nervous system, regulation of emotion, and stress reactivity? *BioPsychoSocial Medicine, 2*, 21.

Harricharan, S., McKinnon, M. C., & Lanius, R. A. (2021). How processing of sensory information from the internal and external worlds shape the perception and engagement with the world in the aftermath of trauma: Implications for PTSD. *Frontiers in Neuroscience, 15*, 625490.

Harricharan, S., McKinnon, M. C., Tursich, M., Densmore, M., Frewen, P., Theberge, J., et al. (2019). Overlapping frontoparietal networks in response to oculomotion and traumatic autobiographical memory retrieval: Implications for eye movement desensitization and reprocessing. *European Journal of Psychotraumatology, 10*(1), 1586265.

Harricharan, S., Nicholson, A. A., Densmore, M., Theberge, J., McKinnon, M. C., Neufeld, R. W. J., et al. (2017). Sensory overload and imbalance: Resting-state vestibular connectivity in PTSD and its dissociative subtype. *Neuropsychologia, 106*, 169–178.

Harricharan, S., Nicholson, A. A., Thome, J., Densmore, M., McKinnon, M. C., Theberge, J., et al. (2020). PTSD and its dissociative subtype through the lens of the insula: Anterior and posterior insula resting-state functional connectivity and its predictive validity using machine learning. *Psychophysiology, 57*(1), e13472.

Harricharan, S., Rabellino, D., Frewen, P. A., Densmore, M., Theberge, J., McKinnon, M. C., et al. (2016). fMRI functional connectivity of the periaqueductal gray in PTSD and its dissociative subtype. *Brain and Behavior, 6*(12), e00579.

Harris, L. R. (2011). Visual and proprioceptive contributions to the perception of one's body. *I-Perception, 2*(8), 885.

Heba, S., Lenz, M., Kalisch, T., Hoffken, O., Schweizer, L. M., Glaubitz, B., et al. (2017). Regionally specific regulation of sensorimotor network connectivity following tactile improvement. *Neural Plasticity, 2017*, 5270532.

Hebb, D. O. (2002). *The organization of behavior: A neuropsychological theory.* Wiley.

Heim, N., Bobou, M., Tanzer, M., Jenkinson, P. M., Steinert, C., & Fotopoulou, A. (2023). Psychological interventions for interoception in mental health disorders: A systematic review of randomized-controlled trials. *Psychiatry and Clinical Neurosciences, 77*(10), 530–540.

Herculano-Houzel, S. (2009). The human brain in numbers: A linearly scaled-up primate brain. *Frontiers in Human Neuroscience, 3*, 857.

Herman, J. L. (1992a). Complex PTSD: A syndrome in survivors of prolonged and repeated trauma. *Journal of Traumatic Stress, 5*(3), 377–391.

Herman, J. L. (1992b). *Trauma and recovery.* Basic Books.

Herman, J. L. (2015). *Trauma and recovery: The aftermath of violence—From domestic abuse to political terror.* Basic Books.

Herman, J. L. (2023). *Truth and repair: How trauma survivors envision justice.* Basic Books.

Hesse, E., & Main, M. (2000). Disorganized infant, child, and adult attachment: Collapse in behavioral and attentional strategies. *Journal of the American Psychoanalytic Association, 48*(4), 1097–1127; discussion 1175–1087.

Holmes, S. E., Scheinost, D., DellaGioia, N., Davis, M. T., Matuskey, D., Pietrzak, R. H., et al. (2018). Cerebellar and prefrontal cortical alterations in PTSD: Structural and functional evidence. *Chronic Stress, 2.*

Horn, A. K. (2006). The reticular formation. *Progress in Brain Research, 151*, 127–155.

Hötting, K., Schickert, N., Kaiser, J., Röder, B., & Schmidt-Kassow, M. (2016). The effects of acute physical exercise on memory, peripheral BDNF, and cortisol in young adults. *Neural Plasticity, 2016*, 6860573.

Hubel, D. H., & Wiesel, T. N. (1979). Brain mechanisms of vision. *Scientific American, 241*(3), 150–162.

Ianì, F. (2019). Embodied memories: Reviewing the role of the body in memory processes. *Psychonomic Bulletin and Review, 26*(6), 1747–1766.

Ibitoye, R. T., Mallas, E. J., Bourke, N. J., Kaski, D., Bronstein, A. M., & Sharp, D. J. (2023). The human vestibular cortex: Functional anatomy of OP2, its connectivity and the effect of vestibular disease. *Cerebral Cortex, 33*(3), 567–582.

Ives-Deliperi, V. L., Solms, M., & Meintjes, E. M. (2011). The neural substrates of mindfulness: An fMRI investigation. *Social Neuroscience, 6*(3), 231–242.

Janacsek, K., Evans, T. M., Kiss, M., Shah, L., Blumenfeld, H., & Ullman, M. T. (2022). Subcortical cognition: The fruit below the rind. *Annual Review of Neuroscience, 45*, 361–386.

Janet, P. (1889). *L'automatisme psychologique: Essai de psychologie expérimentale sur les formes inférieures de l'activité humaine.* Ancienne Librairie Germer Bailliere et Cie.

Janet, P., & Prince, M. (1907). A symposium on the subconscious. *Journal of Abnormal Psychology, 2*(2), 58–92.

Jaradeh, S. S., & Prieto, T. E. (2003). Evaluation of the autonomic nervous system. *Physical Medicine and Rehabilitation Clinics of North America, 14*(2), 287–305.

Javanbakht, A., Liberzon, I., Amirsadri, A., Gjini, K., & Boutros, N. N. (2011). Event-related potential studies of post-traumatic stress disorder: A critical review and synthesis. *Biology of Mood and Anxiety Disorders, 1*(1), 5.

Jinkerson, J. D. (2016). Defining and assessing moral injury: A syndrome perspective. *Traumatology, 22*(2), 122–130.

Johnson, E. O., Babis, G. C., Soultanis, K. C., & Soucacos, P. N. (2008). Functional neuro-anatomy of proprioception. *Journal of Surgical Orthopaedic Advances, 17*(3), 159–164.

Kabat-Zinn, J. (2003). Mindfulness-based interventions in context: Past, present, and future. *Clinical Psychology: Science and Practice, 10*(2), 144–156.

Karl, A., Schaefer, M., Malta, L. S., Dorfel, D., Rohleder, N., & Werner, A. (2006). A meta-analysis of structural brain abnormalities in PTSD. *Neuroscience and Biobehavioral Reviews, 30*(7), 1004–1031.

Kavanagh, D. J., Freese, S., Andrade, J., & May, J. (2001). Effects of visuospatial tasks on desensitization to emotive memories. *British Journal of Clinical Psychology, 40*(3), 267–280.

Kaye, A. P., & Krystal, J. H. (2020). Predictive processing in mental illness: Hierarchical circuitry for perception and trauma. *Journal of Abnormal Psychology, 129*(6), 629–632.

Kayser, C., Ince, R. A., & Panzeri, S. (2012). Analysis of slow (theta) oscillations as a potential temporal reference frame for information coding in sensory cortices. *PLoS Computational Biology, 8*(10), e1002717.

Kayser, C., & Logothetis, N. K. (2007). Do early sensory cortices integrate cross-modal information? *Brain Structure and Function, 212*, 121–132.

Kearney, B. E., Corrigan, F. M., Frewen, P. A., Nevill, S., Harricharan, S., Andrews, K., et al. (2023). A randomized controlled trial of deep brain reorienting: A neuroscientifically guided treatment for post-traumatic stress disorder. *European Journal Psychotraumatology, 14*(2), 2240691.

Kearney, B. E., & Lanius, R. A. (2022). The brain–body disconnect: A somatic sensory basis for trauma-related disorders. *Frontiers in Neuroscience, 16*, 1015749.

Kearney, B. E., & Lanius, R. A. (2024). Why reliving is not remembering and the unique neuro-biological representation of traumatic memory. *Nature Mental Health, 2*(10), 1142–1151.

Kearney, B. E., Terpou, B. A., Densmore, M., Shaw, S. B., Theberge, J., Jetly, R., et al. (2023). How the body remembers: Examining the default mode and sensorimotor networks during moral injury autobiographical memory retrieval in PTSD. *NeuroImage: Clinical, 38*, 103426.

Kennis, M., Rademaker, A. R., van Rooij, S. J., Kahn, R. S., & Geuze, E. (2015). Resting state functional connectivity of the anterior cingulate cortex in veterans with and without post-traumatic stress disorder. *Human Brain Mapping, 36*(1), 99–109.

Kerley, L. J., Meredith, P. J., & Harnett, P. H. (2023). The relationship between sensory processing and attachment patterns: A scoping review. *Canadian Journal of Occupational Therapy, 90*(1), 79–91.

Khoury, J. E., Pechtel, P., Andersen, C. M., Teicher, M. H., & Lyons-Ruth, K. (2019). Relations among maternal withdrawal in infancy, borderline features, suicidality/self-injury, and adult hippocampal volume: A 30-year longitudinal study. *Behavioral Brain Research, 374*, 112139.

Kierkegaard, S. (1980). *The sickness unto death* (H. V. Hong & E. H. Hong, Trans.). Princeton University Press. (Original work published 1849)

Kingma, H., & van de Berg, R. (2016). Anatomy, physiology, and physics of the peripheral vestibular system. In *Handbook of clinical neurology* (Vol. 137, pp. 1–16). Elsevier.

Kleim, B., Ehring, T., & Ehlers, A. (2012). Perceptual processing advantages for trauma-related visual cues in post-traumatic stress disorder. *Psychological Medicine, 42*(1), 173–181.

Kluetsch, R. C., Ros, T., Theberge, J., Frewen, P. A., Calhoun, V. D., Schmahl, C., et al. (2014). Plastic modulation of PTSD resting-state networks and subjective wellbeing by EEG neurofeedback. *Acta Psychiatrica Scandinavica, 130*(2), 123–136.

Kluft, R. P. (1990). On the apparent invisibility of incest: A personal reflection on things known and forgotten. In R. P. Kluft (Ed.), *Incest-related syndromes of adult psychopathology* (pp. 11–34). American Psychiatric Association.

Kluft, R. P. (1993). The initial stages of psychotherapy in the treatment of multiple personality disorder patients. *Dissociation: Progress in the Dissociative Disorders, 6*(2–3), 145–161.

Koch, C., Massimini, M., Boly, M., & Tononi, G. (2016). Neural correlates of consciousness: Progress and problems. *Nature Reviews Neuroscience, 17*(5), 307–321.

Kozlowska, K., Walker, P., McLean, L., & Carrive, P. (2015). Fear and the defense cascade: Clinical implications and management. *Harvard Review of Psychiatry, 23*(4), 263–287.

Kropf, E., Syan, S. K., Minuzzi, L., & Frey, B. N. (2019). From anatomy to function: The role of the somatosensory cortex in emotional regulation. *Brazilian Journal of Psychiatry, 41*(3), 261–269.

Krystal, H. (1988). *Integration and self healing: Affect, trauma, alexithymia.* Routledge.

Krystal, J. H., Bennett, A. L., Bremner, J. D., Southwick, S. M., Charney, D. S. (1995). Toward a cognitive neuroscience of dissociation and altered memory functions in post-traumatic stress disorder. In M. J. Friedman, D. S. Charney, & A. Y. Deutsch (Eds.), *Neurobiological and clinical consequences of stress: From normal adaptions to PTSD* (pp 239–268). Raven Press

Kuhfuß, M., Maldei, T., Hetmanek, A., & Baumann, N. (2021). Somatic experiencing—Effectiveness and key factors of a body-oriented trauma therapy: A scoping literature review. *European Journal of Psychotraumatology, 12*(1), 1929023.

Lacquaniti, F., Bosco, G., Gravano, S., Indovina, I., La Scaleia, B., Maffei, V., et al. (2014). Multisensory integration and internal models for sensing gravity effects in primates. *BioMed Research International, 2014,* 615854.

Lamb, D. G., Porges, E. C., Lewis, G. F., & Williamson, J. B. (2017). Non-invasive vagal nerve stimulation effects on hyperarousal and autonomic state in patients with posttraumatic stress disorder and history of mild traumatic brain injury: Preliminary evidence. *Frontiers in Medicine, 4,* 124.

Landin-Romero, R., Moreno-Alcazar, A., Pagani, M., & Amann, B. L. (2018). How does eye movement desensitization and reprocessing therapy work?: A systematic review on suggested mechanisms of action. *Frontiers in Psychology, 9,* 286360.

Lane, S. J., Mailloux, Z., Schoen, S., Bundy, A., May-Benson, T. A., Parham, L. D., et al. (2019). Neural foundations of Ayres Sensory Integration®. *Brain Sciences, 9*(7), 153.

Langmuir, J. I., Kirsh, S. G., & Classen, C. C. (2012). A pilot study of body-oriented group psychotherapy: Adapting sensorimotor psychotherapy for the group treatment of trauma. *Psychological Trauma: Theory, Research, Practice, and Policy, 4*(2), 214–220.

Lanius, R. A., Boyd, J. E., McKinnon, M. C., Nicholson, A. A., Frewen, P., Vermetten, E., et al. (2018). A review of the neurobiological basis of trauma-related dissociation and its relation to cannabinoid- and opioid-mediated stress response: A transdiagnostic, translational approach. *Current Psychiatry Reports, 20*(12), 118.

Lanius, R. A., Frewen, P. A., Tursich, M., Jetly, R., & McKinnon, M. C. (2015). Restoring large-scale brain networks in PTSD and related disorders: A proposal for neuroscientifically-informed treatment interventions. *European Journal of Psychotraumatology, 6*(1), 1–12.

Lanius, R. A., Hopper, J. W., & Menon, R. S. (2003). Individual differences in a husband and wife who developed PTSD after a motor vehicle accident: A functional MRI case study. *American Journal of Psychiatry, 160*(4), 667–669.

Lanius, R. A., Rabellino, D., Boyd, J. E., Harricharan, S., Frewen, P. A., & McKinnon, M. C. (2017). The innate alarm system in PTSD: Conscious and subconscious processing of threat. *Current Opinions in Psychology, 14,* 109–115.

Lanius, R. A., Terpou, B. A., & McKinnon, M. C. (2020). The sense of self in the aftermath of trauma: Lessons from the default mode network in posttraumatic stress disorder. *European Journal of Psychotraumatology, 11*(1), 1807703.

Lanius, R. A., Vermetten, E., Loewenstein, R. J., Brand, B., Schmahl, C., Bremner, J. D., et al. (2010). Emotion modulation in PTSD: Clinical and neurobiological evidence for a dissociative subtype. *American Journal of Psychiatry, 167*(6), 640–647.

Lanius, U. F., Paulsen, S. L., & Corrigan, F. M. (2014). *Neurobiology and treatment of traumatic dissociation: Towards an embodied self.* Springer.

Lavoisier, A. L. (1789). *Traité élémentaire de chimie* (Vol. 1). Chez Cuchet.

Lebel, C., Walker, L., Leemans, A., Phillips, L., & Beaulieu, C. (2008). Microstructural maturation of the human brain from childhood to adulthood. *NeuroImage, 40*(3), 1044–1055.

Lebois, L. A. M., Seligowski, A. V., Wolff, J. D., Hill, S. B., & Ressler, K. J. (2019). Augmentation of extinction and inhibitory learning in anxiety and trauma-related disorders. *Annual Review of Clinical Psychology, 15*(1), 257–284.

LeDoux, J. (2003). The emotional brain, fear, and the amygdala. *Cellular and Molecular Neurobiology, 23*(4–5), 727–738.

Lentini, J. A., & Knox, M. S. (2015). Equine-facilitated psychotherapy with children and adolescents: An update and literature review. *Journal of Creativity in Mental Health, 10*(3), 278–305.

Levine, P. A. (2010). *In an unspoken voice: How the body releases trauma and restores goodness.* North Atlantic Books.

Levit-Binnun, N., Szepsenwol, O., Stern-Ellran, K., & Engel-Yeger, B. (2014). The relationship between sensory responsiveness profiles, attachment orientations, and anxiety symptoms. *Australian Journal of Psychology, 66*(4), 233–240.

Linden, D. J. (2016). *Touch: The science of hand, heart and mind.* Penguin Books.

Lindquist, K. A., Wager, T. D., Kober, H., Bliss-Moreau, E., & Barrett, L. F. (2012). The brain basis of emotion: A meta-analytic review. *Behavioral and Brain Sciences, 35*(3), 121–143.

Linehan, M. (1993). *Skills training manual for treating borderline personality disorder.* Guilford Press.

Linehan, M. (2014). *DBT skills training manual* (2nd ed.). Guilford Press.

Litz, B. T., & Gray, M. J. (2002). Emotional numbing in posttraumatic stress disorder: Current and future research directions. *Australian and New Zealand Journal of Psychiatry, 36*(2), 198–204.

Litz, B. T., Stein, N., Delaney, E., Lebowitz, L., Nash, W. P., Silva, C., et al. (2009). Moral injury and moral repair in war veterans: A preliminary model and intervention strategy. *Clinical Psychological Review, 29*(8), 695–706.

Lloyd, C. S., Lanius, R. A., Brown, M. F., Neufeld, R. J., Frewen, P. A., & McKinnon, M. C. (2019). Assessing post-traumatic tonic immobility responses: The scale for tonic immobility occurring post-trauma. *Chronic Stress, 3*, 2470547018822492.

Lloyd, C. S., Nicholson, A. A., Densmore, M., Theberge, J., Neufeld, R. W. J., Jetly, R., et al. (2021). Shame on the brain: Neural correlates of moral injury event recall in posttraumatic stress disorder. *Depression and Anxiety, 38*(6), 596–605.

Loewald, H. W. (1971). Some considerations on repetition and repetition compulsion. *International Journal of Psychoanalysis, 52*(1), 59–66.

Lopez, C., & Blanke, O. (2011). The thalamocortical vestibular system in animals and humans. *Brain Research Reviews, 67*(1–2), 119–146.

Lopez, C., Halje, P., & Blanke, O. (2008). Body ownership and embodiment: Vestibular and multisensory mechanisms. *Neurophysiologie Clinique/Clinical Neurophysiology, 38*(3), 149–161.

Lux, V., Non, A. L., Pexman, P. M., Stadler, W., Weber, L. A. E., & Kruger, M. (2021). A developmental framework for embodiment research: The next step toward integrating concepts and methods. *Frontiers in Systematic Neuroscience, 15*, 672740.

Lyons-Ruth, K. (2003). Dissociation and the parent–infant dialogue: A longitudinal perspective from attachment research. *Journal of the American Psychoanalytic Association, 51*(3), 883–911.

Lyons-Ruth, K. (2007). The interface between attachment and intersubjectivity: Perspective from the longitudinal study of disorganized attachment. *Psychoanalytic Inquiry, 26*(4), 595–616.

Lyons-Ruth, K., & Block, D. (1996). The disturbed caregiving system: Relations among childhood trauma, maternal caregiving, and infant affect and attachment. *Infant Mental Health Journal, 17*(3), 257–275.

Lyons-Ruth, K., & Yarger, H. A. (2022). Developmental costs associated with early maternal withdrawal. *Child Development Perspectives, 16*(1), 10–17.

MacLean, P. D. (1990). *The triune brain in evolution: Role in paleocerebral functions.* Springer Science & Business Media.

Magoun, H. W. (1952). An ascending reticular activating system in the brain stem. *A.M.A. Archives of Neurology and Psychiatry, 67*(2), 145–154; discussion 167–171.

Maier, A., Heinen-Ludwig, L., Gunturkun, O., Hurlemann, R., & Scheele, D. (2020). Childhood maltreatment alters the neural processing of chemosensory stress signals. *Frontiers in Psychiatry, 11,* 783.

Maier, J. X., Chandrasekaran, C., & Ghazanfar, A. A. (2008). Integration of bimodal looming signals through neuronal coherence in the temporal lobe. *Current Biology, 18*(13), 963–968.

Makino, S., Hashimoto, K., & Gold, P. W. (2002). Multiple feedback mechanisms activating corticotropin-releasing hormone system in the brain during stress. *Pharmacology, Biochemistry, and Behavior, 73*(1), 147–158.

Malchiodi, C. A. (2020). *Trauma and expressive arts therapy: Brain, body, and imagination in the healing process.* Guilford Press.

Malchiodi, C. A. (2022). *Handbook of expressive arts therapy.* Guilford Press.

Malejko, K., Abler, B., Plener, P. L., & Straub, J. (2017). Neural correlates of psychotherapeutic treatment of post-traumatic stress disorder: A systematic literature review. *Frontiers in Psychiatry, 8,* 85.

Marshall, A. C., Gentsch, A., & Schutz-Bosbach, S. (2018). The interaction between interoceptive and action states within a framework of predictive coding. *Frontiers in Psychology, 9,* 180.

Martins, I., & Tavares, I. (2017). Reticular formation and pain: The past and the future. *Frontiers in Neuroanatomy, 11,* 51.

Mast, F. W., Merfeld, D. M., & Kosslyn, S. M. (2006). Visual mental imagery during caloric vestibular stimulation. *Neuropsychologia, 44*(1), 101–109.

Maté, G. (2010). *In the realm of hungry ghosts: Close encounters with addiction.* North Atlantic Books.

Maté, G. (2011). *When the body says no: The cost of hidden stress.* Vintage Canada.

Maté, G., & Maté, D. (2022). *The myth of normal: Trauma, illness and healing in a toxic culture.* Ebury.

Maxfield, L., Melnyk, W. T., & Hayman, G. C. (2008). A working memory explanation for the effects of eye movements in EMDR. *Journal of EMDR Practice and Research, 2*(4), 247–261.

McCarthy, G., Puce, A., Gore, J. C., & Allison, T. (1997). Face-specific processing in the human fusiform gyrus. *Journal of Cognitive Neuroscience, 9*(5), 605–610.

McCorry, L. K. (2007). Physiology of the autonomic nervous system. *American Journal of Pharmaceutical Education, 71*(4), 78.

McCullough, L., Risley-Curtiss, C., & Rorke, J. (2015). Equine facilitated psychotherapy: A pilot study of effect on posttraumatic stress symptoms in maltreated youth. *Journal of Infant, Child and Adolescent Psychotherapy, 14*(2), 158–173.

McEwen, B. S. (2013). The brain on stress: Toward an integrative approach to brain, body, and behavior. *Perspectives on Psychological Science, 8*(6), 673–675.

McGlone, F., Wessberg, J., & Olausson, H. (2014). Discriminative and affective touch: Sensing and feeling. *Neuron, 82*(4), 737–755.

Menon, V. (2011). Large-scale brain networks and psychopathology: A unifying triple network model. *Trends in Cognitive Sciences, 15*(10), 483–506.

Milad, M. R., Pitman, R. K., Ellis, C. B., Gold, A. L., Shin, L. M., Lasko, N. B., et al. (2009). Neurobiological basis of failure to recall extinction memory in posttraumatic stress disorder. *Biological Psychiatry, 66*(12), 1075–1082.

Miller, D. R., Hayes, S. M., Hayes, J. P., Spielberg, J. M., Lafleche, G., & Verfaellie, M. (2017). Default mode network subsystems are differentially disrupted in posttraumatic stress disorder. *Biological Psychiatry: Cognitive Neuroscience and Neuroimaging, 2*(4), 363–371.

Mithoefer, M. C., Grob, C. S., & Brewerton, T. D. (2016). Novel psychopharmacological therapies for psychiatric disorders: Psilocybin and MDMA. *Lancet Psychiatry, 3*(5), 481–488.

Mobbs, D., Marchant, J. L., Hassabis, D., Seymour, B., Tan, G., Gray, M., et al. (2009). From threat to fear: The neural organization of defensive fear systems in humans. *Journal of Neuroscience, 29*(39), 12236–12243.

Mobbs, D., Petrovic, P., Marchant, J. L., Hassabis, D., Weiskopf, N., Seymour, B., et al. (2007). When fear is near: Threat imminence elicits prefrontal–periaqueductal gray shifts in humans. *Science, 317*, 1079–1083.

Moll, J., de Oliveira-Souza, R., Moll, F. T., Ignacio, F. A., Bramati, I. E., Caparelli-Daquer, E. M., et al. (2005). The moral affiliations of disgust: A functional MRI study. *Cognitive and Behavioral Neurology, 18*(1), 68–78.

Mombaerts, P. (2001). How smell develops. *Nature Neuroscience, 4*, 1192–1198.

Mueller, M. K., & McCullough, L. (2017). Effects of equine-facilitated psychotherapy on posttraumatic stress symptoms in youth. *Journal of Child and Family Studies, 26*(4), 1164–1172.

Mullen, B., Champagne, T., Krishnamurty, S., Dickson, D., & Gao, R. X. (2008). Exploring the safety and therapeutic effects of deep pressure stimulation using a weighted blanket. *Occupational Therapy in Mental Health, 24*(1), 65–89.

Muret, D., Root, V., Kieliba, P., Clode, D., & Makin, T. R. (2022). Beyond body maps: Information content of specific body parts is distributed across the somatosensory homunculus. *Cell Reports, 38*(11), 110523.

Murkar, A. L. A., & De Koninck, J. (2018). Consolidative mechanisms of emotional processing in REM sleep and PTSD. *Sleep Medicine Reviews, 41*, 173–184.

Murray, M. M., Thelen, A., Thut, G., Romei, V., Martuzzi, R., & Matusz, P. J. (2016). The multisensory function of the human primary visual cortex. *Neuropsychologia, 83*, 161–169.

Myrick, A. C., Webermann, A. R., Loewenstein, R. J., Lanius, R., Putnam, F. W., & Brand, B. L. (2017). Six-year follow-up of the treatment of patients with dissociative disorders study. *European Journal of Psychotraumatology, 8*(1), 1344080.

Nakazawa, D. J. (2015). *Childhood disrupted: How your biography becomes your biology, and how you can heal.* Simon & Schuster.

Nakazawa, D. J. (2021). *The angel and the assassin: The tiny brain cell that changed the course of medicine.* Random House.

Namkung, H., Kim, S. H., & Sawa, A. (2017). The insula: An underestimated brain area in clinical neuroscience, psychiatry, and neurology. *Trends in Neuroscience, 40*(4), 200–207.

Naste, T. M., Price, M., Karol, J., Martin, L., Murphy, K., Miguel, J., et al. (2018). Equine facilitated therapy for complex trauma (EFT-CT). *Journal of Child and Adolescent Trauma, 11*(3), 289–303.

Nauta, W. J., & Feirtag, M. (1979). The organization of the brain. *Scientific American, 241*(3), 88–111.

Ndubuizu, O., & LaManna, J. C. (2007). Brain tissue oxygen concentration measurements. *Antioxidants and Redox Signaling, 9*(8), 1207–1219.

Nicholson, A. A., Friston, K. J., Zeidman, P., Harricharan, S., McKinnon, M. C., Densmore, M., et al. (2017). Dynamic causal modeling in PTSD and its dissociative subtype: Bottom-up versus top-down processing within fear and emotion regulation circuitry. *Human Brain Mapping, 38*(11), 5551–5561.

Nicholson, A. A., Rabellino, D., Densmore, M., Frewen, P. A., Paret, C., Kluetsch, R., et al. (2018). Intrinsic connectivity network dynamics in PTSD during amygdala downregulation using real-time fMRI neurofeedback: A preliminary analysis. *Human Brain Mapping, 39*(11), 4258–4275.

Nicholson, A. A., Ros, T., Densmore, M., Frewen, P. A., Neufeld, R. W. J., Theberge, J., et al. (2020). A randomized, controlled trial of alpha-rhythm EEG neurofeedback in posttraumatic stress disorder: A preliminary investigation showing evidence of decreased PTSD symptoms and restored default mode and salience network connectivity using fMRI. *NeuroImage: Clinical, 28*, 102490.

Nicholson, A. A., Sapru, I., Densmore, M., Frewen, P. A., Neufeld, R. W., Theberge, J., et al. (2016). Unique insula subregion resting-state functional connectivity with amygdala complexes in posttraumatic stress disorder and its dissociative subtype. *Psychiatry Research: Neuroimaging, 250*, 61–72.

Nin, A. (1961). *Seduction of the minotaur.* Swallow Press.

Norte, C. E., Volchan, E., Vila, J., Mata, J. L., Arbol, J. R., Mendlowicz, M., et al. (2019). Tonic immobility in PTSD: Exacerbation of emotional cardiac defense response. *Frontiers in Psychology, 10*, 1213.

Ogden, P., & Fisher, J. (2015). *Sensorimotor psychotherapy.* Norton.

Ogden, P., Pain, C., & Fisher, J. (2006). A sensorimotor approach to the treatment of trauma and dissociation. *Psychiatric Clinics of North America, 29*(1), 263–279.

Oka, T. (2015). Psychogenic fever: How psychological stress affects body temperature in the clinical population. *Temperature, 2*(3), 368–378.

Oka, T., & Oka, K. (2012). Mechanisms of psychogenic fever. *Advances in Neuroimmune Biology, 3*(1), 3–17.

Olausson, H., Wessberg, J., Morrison, I., McGlone, F., & Vallbo, A. (2010). The neurophysiology of unmyelinated tactile afferents. *Neuroscience and Biobehavioral Reviews, 34*(2), 185–191.

Olive, I., Tempelmann, C., Berthoz, A., & Heinze, H. J. (2015). Increased functional connectivity between superior colliculus and brain regions implicated in bodily self-consciousness during the rubber hand illusion. *Human Brain Mapping, 36*(2), 717–730.

Ortega-de San Luis, C., Pezzoli, M., Urrieta, E., & Ryan, T. J. (2023). Engram cell connectivity as a mechanism for information encoding and memory function. *Current Biology, 33*(24), 5368–5380.

Overmier, J. B., & Seligman, M. E. (1967). Effects of inescapable shock upon subsequent escape and avoidance responding. *Journal of Comparative and Physiological Psychology, 63*(1), 28–33.

Owens, A. P., Allen, M., Ondobaka, S., & Friston, K. J. (2018). Interoceptive inference: From computational neuroscience to clinic. *Neuroscience and Biobehavioral Reviews, 90*, 174–183.

Paciorek, A., & Skora, L. (2020). Vagus nerve stimulation as a gateway to interoception. *Frontiers in Psychology, 11*, 1659.

Pagani, M., Högberg, G., Fernandez, I., & Siracusano, A. (2013). Correlates of EMDR therapy in functional and structural neuroimaging: A critical summary of recent findings. *Journal of EMDR Practice and Research, 7*(1), 29–38.

Palomar-Ciria, N., & Bello, H. J. (2023). Equine-assisted therapy in post-traumatic-stress disorder: A systematic review and meta-analysis. *Journal of Equine Veterinary Science, 128*, 104871.

Panksepp, J. (1998). The periconscious substrates of consciousness: Affective states and the evolutionary origins of the self. *Journal of Consciousness Studies, 5*(5–6), 566–582.

Panksepp, J. (2004). *Affective neuroscience: The foundations of human and animal emotions.* Oxford University Press.

Panksepp, J. (2005). Affective consciousness: Core emotional feelings in animals and humans. *Consciousness and Cognition, 14*(1), 30–80.

Panksepp, J., & Biven, L. (2012). *The archaeology of mind: Neuroevolutionary origins of human emotions.* Norton.

Paulus, M. P., & Stein, M. B. (2010). Interoception in anxiety and depression. *Brain Structure and Function, 214*(5–6), 451–463.

Payne, P., Levine, P. A., & Crane-Godreau, M. A. (2015). Somatic experiencing: Using interoception and proprioception as core elements of trauma therapy. *Frontiers in Psychology, 6*, 93.

Peever, J., & Fuller, P. M. (2017). The biology of REM sleep. *Current Biology, 27*(22), R1237–R1248.

Pellegrino, R., Farruggia, M. C., Small, D. M., & Veldhuizen, M. G. (2021). Post-traumatic olfactory loss and brain response beyond olfactory cortex. *Scientific Reports, 11*(1), 4043.

Perl, O., Duek, O., Kulkarni, K. R., Gordon, C., Krystal, J. H., Levy, I., et al. (2023). Neural patterns differentiate traumatic from sad autobiographical memories in PTSD. *Nature Neuroscience, 26*(12), 2226–2236.

Perry, B. D. (2019). The neurosequential model: A developmentally sensitive, neuroscience-informed approach to clinical problem-solving. In J. Mitchell, J. Tucci, & E. Tronick (Eds.), *The handbook of therapeutic care for children: Evidence informed approaches to working with traumatized children and adolescents in foster, kinship and adoptive care* (pp. 137–158). Jessica Kingsley.

Pfeiffer, C., Serino, A., & Blanke, O. (2014). The vestibular system: A spatial reference for bodily self-consciousness. *Frontiers in Integrative Neuroscience, 8*, 31.

Piaget, J. (1962). The relation of affectivity to intelligence in the mental development of the child. *Bulletin of the Menninger Clinic, 26*(3), 129–137.

Pitman, R. K., van der Kolk, B. A., Orr, S. P., & Greenberg, M. S. (1990). Naloxone-reversible analgesic response to combat-related stimuli in posttraumatic stress disorder: A pilot study. *Archives of General Psychiatry, 47*(6), 541–544.

Platt, M. G., & Freyd, J. J. (2015). Betray my trust, shame on me: Shame, dissociation, fear, and betrayal trauma. *Psychological Trauma: Theory, Research, Practice, and Policy, 7*(4), 398–404.

Ploner, M., Schmitz, F., Freund, H. J., & Schnitzler, A. (2000). Differential organization of touch and pain in human primary somatosensory cortex. *Journal of Neurophysiology, 83*(3), 1770–1776.

Poppenk, J., & Moscovitch, M. (2011). A hippocampal marker of recollection memory ability among healthy young adults: Contributions of posterior and anterior segments. *Neuron, 72*(6), 931–937.

Porges, S. W., & Rossetti, A. (2018). Music, music therapy and trauma. *Music and Medicine, 10*(3), 117–120.

Preusser, S., Thiel, S. D., Rook, C., Roggenhofer, E., Kosatschek, A., Draganski, B., et al. (2015). The perception of touch and the ventral somatosensory pathway. *Brain, 138*(Pt. 3), 540–548.

Putnam, F. W. (1989). Pierre Janet and modern views of dissociation. *Journal of Traumatic Stress, 2*(4), 413–429.

Qin, L. D., Wang, Z., Sun, Y. W., Wan, J. Q., Su, S. S., Zhou, Y., et al. (2012). A preliminary study of alterations in default network connectivity in post-traumatic stress disorder patients following recent trauma. *Brain Research, 1484*, 50–56.

Qin, P., & Northoff, G. (2011). How is our self related to midline regions and the default-mode network? *NeuroImage, 57*(3), 1221–1233.

Quak, M., London, R. E., & Talsma, D. (2015). A multisensory perspective of working memory. *Frontiers in Human Neuroscience, 9*, 197.

Quigley, K. S., Kanoski, S., Grill, W. M., Barrett, L. F., & Tsakiris, M. (2021). Functions of interoception: From energy regulation to experience of the self. *Trends in Neuroscience, 44*(1), 29–38.

Rabellino, D., Thome, J., Densmore, M., Theberge, J., McKinnon, M. C., & Lanius, R. A. (2023). The vestibulocerebellum and the shattered self: A resting-state functional connectivity study in posttraumatic stress disorder and its dissociative subtype. *Cerebellum, 22*(6), 1083–1097.

Rachman, S. (1980). Emotional processing. *Behaviour Research Therapy, 18*(1), 51–60.

Raichle, M. E., & Gusnard, D. A. (2002). Appraising the brain's energy budget. *Proceedings of the National Academy of Sciences of the United States of America, 99*(16), 10237–10239.

Resick, P. A., Monson, C. M., & Chard, K. M. (2017). *Cognitive processing therapy for PTSD: A comprehensive manual.* Guilford Press.

Resick, P. A., Monson, C. M., & Chard, K. M. (2024). *Cognitive processing therapy for PTSD: A comprehensive therapist manual* (2nd ed.). Guilford Press.

Richter-Levin, G., & Akirav, I. (2000). Amygdala–hippocampus dynamic interaction in relation to memory. *Molecular Neurobiology, 22*(1–3), 11–20.

Robinson, T. E., & Berridge, K. C. (2008). The incentive sensitization theory of addiction: Some current issues. *Philosophical Transactions of the Royal Society. B: Biological Sciences, 363,* 3137–3146.

Rodwin, A. H., Shimizu, R., Travis, R., Jr., James, K. J., Banya, M., & Munson, M. R. (2023). A systematic review of music-based interventions to improve treatment engagement and mental health outcomes for adolescents and young adults. *Child and Adolescent Social Work Journal, 40*(4), 537–566.

Rolls, E. T. (2019). The cingulate cortex and limbic systems for emotion, action, and memory. *Brain Structure and Function, 224*(9), 3001–3018.

Rothbaum, B. O., & Schwartz, A. C. (2002). Exposure therapy for posttraumatic stress disorder. *American Journal of Psychotherapy, 56*(1), 59–75.

Rothschild, B. (2000). *The body remembers: The psychophysiology of trauma and trauma treatment.* Norton.

Rothschild, B. (2017). *The body remembers: Vol. 2. Revolutionizing trauma treatment.* Norton.

Rothschild, G. (2019). The transformation of multi-sensory experiences into memories during sleep. *Neurobiology of Learning and Memory, 160,* 58–66.

Rousseau, P. F., El Khoury-Malhame, M., Reynaud, E., Zendjidjian, X., Samuelian, J. C., & Khalfa, S. (2019). Neurobiological correlates of EMDR therapy effect in PTSD. *European Journal of Trauma and Dissociation, 3*(2), 103–111.

Routtenberg, A. (1968). The two-arousal hypothesis: Reticular formation and limbic system. *Psychological Review, 75*(1), 51–80.

Roux, F. E., Djidjeli, I., & Durand, J. B. (2018). Functional architecture of the somatosensory homunculus detected by electrostimulation. *Journal of Physiology, 596*(5), 941–956.

Santaella, D. F., Balardin, J. B., Afonso, R. F., Giorjiani, G. M., Sato, J. R., Lacerda, S. S., et al. (2019). Greater anteroposterior default mode network functional connectivity in long-term elderly yoga practitioners. *Frontiers in Aging Neuroscience, 11,* 158.

Sapolsky, R. M. (2015). Stress and the brain: Individual variability and the inverted-U. *Nature Neuroscience, 18*(10), 1344–1346.

Scaravelli, V. (1991). *Awakening the spine: The stress-free new yoga that works with the body to restore health, vitality and energy.* HarperOne.

Schaefer, M., Kuhnel, A., Schweitzer, F., Rumpel, F., & Gartner, M. (2023). Experiencing sweet taste is associated with an increase in prosocial behavior. *Scientific Reports, 13*(1), 1954.

Schauer, M., & Elbert, T. (2010). Dissociation following traumatic stress: Etiology and treatment. *Journal of Psychology, 218*(2), 109–127.

Schiavone, F. L., Frewen, P., McKinnon, M., & Lanius, R. A. (2018). The dissociative subtype of PTSD: An update of the literature. *PTSD Research Quarterly, 29*(3), 1–13.

Schore, A. N. (2003). *Affect dysregulation and disorders of the self.* Norton.

Schore, J. R., & Schore, A. N. (2008). Modern attachment theory: The central role of affect regulation in development and treatment. *Clinical Social Work Journal, 36*(1), 9–20.

Schouten, K. A., de Niet, G. J., Knipscheer, J. W., Kleber, R. J., & Hutschemaekers, G. J. (2015). The effectiveness of art therapy in the treatment of traumatized adults: A systematic review on art therapy and trauma. *Trauma, Violence and Abuse, 16*(2), 220–228.

Schulz, A., Schultchen, D., & Vögele, C. (2020). Interoception, stress, and physical symptoms in stress-associated diseases. *European Journal of Health Psychology, 27*(4), 132–153.

Schulz, A., & Vogele, C. (2015). Interoception and stress. *Frontiers in Psychology, 6,* 993.

Seeley, W. W., Menon, V., Schatzberg, A. F., Keller, J., Glover, G. H., Kenna, H., et al. (2007). Dissociable intrinsic connectivity networks for salience processing and executive control. *Journal of Neuroscience, 27*(9), 2349–2356.

Segal, Z., Williams, M., & Teasdale, J. (2018). *Mindfulness-based cognitive therapy for depression* (2nd ed.). Guilford Press.

Seligman, M. E. (1972). Learned helplessness. *Annual Review of Medicine, 23,* 407–412.

Selye, H. (1950). Stress and the general adaptation syndrome. *British Medical Journal, 1*(4667), 1383–1392.

Seth, A. K., & Friston, K. J. (2016). Active interoceptive inference and the emotional brain. *Philosophical Transactions of the Royal Society. Series B: Biological Sciences 371*(1708).

Seth, A. K., Suzuki, K., & Critchley, H. D. (2012). An interoceptive predictive coding model of conscious presence. *Frontiers in Psychology, 2,* 395.

Shaffer, J. (2016). Neuroplasticity and clinical practice: Building brain power for health. *Frontiers in Psychology, 7,* 1118.

Shams, L., & Seitz, A. R. (2008). Benefits of multisensory learning. *Trends in Cognitive Sciences, 12*(11), 411–417.

Shang, J., Lui, S., Meng, Y., Zhu, H., Qiu, C., Gong, Q., et al. (2014). Alterations in low-level perceptual networks related to clinical severity in PTSD after an earthquake: A resting-state fMRI study. *PLoS One, 9*(5), e96834.

Shapiro, F. (1989). Eye movement desensitization: A new treatment for post-traumatic stress disorder. *Journal of Behavior Therapy and Experimental Psychiatry, 20*(3), 211–217.

Shapiro, F., & Maxfield, L. (2002). Eye movement desensitization and reprocessing (EMDR): Information processing in the treatment of trauma. *Journal of Clinical Psychology, 58*(8), 933–946.

Shapiro, L. (2014). *The Routledge handbook of embodied cognition.* Routledge.

Shields, M., Tonmyr, L., Hovdestad, W. E., Gonzalez, A., & MacMillan, H. (2020). Exposure to family violence from childhood to adulthood. *BMC Public Health, 20*(1), 1673.

Shine, J. M., Breakspear, M., Bell, P. T., Ehgoetz Martens, K. A., Shine, R., Koyejo, O., et al. (2019). Human cognition involves the dynamic integration of neural activity and neuro-modulatory systems. *Nature Neuroscience, 22*(2), 289–296.

Siegel, D. (1999). *The developing mind: Toward a neurobiology of interpersonal experience.* Guilford Press.

Siegel, D. J. (2001). Toward an interpersonal neurobiology of the developing mind: Attachment relationships, mindsight, and neural integration: Contributions from the decade of the brain to infant mental health. *Infant Mental Health Journal, 22*(1–2), 67–94.

Siegel, D. J. (2009). Mindful awareness, mindsight, and neural integration. *The Humanistic Psychologist, 37*(2), 137–158.

Siegel, D. J. (2010). *The mindful therapist: A clinician's guide to mindsight and neural integration.* Norton.

Siegel, D. J. (2020). *The developing mind: How relationships and the brain interact to shape who we are* (3rd ed.). Guilford Press.

Siegelaar, S. E., Olff, M., Bour, L. J., Veelo, D., Zwinderman, A. H., van Bruggen, G., et al. (2006). The auditory startle response in post-traumatic stress disorder. *Experimental Brain Research, 174*(1), 1–6.

Simmons, W. K., Avery, J. A., Barcalow, J. C., Bodurka, J., Drevets, W. C., & Bellgowan, P. (2013). Keeping the body in mind: Insula functional organization and functional connectivity integrate interoceptive, exteroceptive, and emotional awareness. *Human Brain Mapping, 34*(11), 2944–2958.

Skora, L. I., Livermore, J. J. A., & Roelofs, K. (2022). The functional role of cardiac activity in perception and action. *Neuroscience and Biobehavioral Reviews, 137,* 104655.

Smith, P. F. (1997). Vestibular–hippocampal interactions. *Hippocampus, 7*(5), 465–471.

Spreng, R. N., & Grady, C. L. (2010). Patterns of brain activity supporting autobiographical memory, prospection, and theory of mind, and their relationship to the default mode network. *Journal of Cognitive Neuroscience, 22*(6), 1112–1123.

Spreng, R. N., Mar, R. A., & Kim, A. S. (2009). The common neural basis of autobiographical memory, prospection, navigation, theory of mind, and the default mode: A quantitative meta-analysis. *Journal of Cognitive Neuroscience, 21*(3), 489–510.

Sripada, R. K., King, A. P., Welsh, R. C., Garfinkel, S. N., Wang, X., Sripada, C. S., et al. (2012). Neural dysregulation in posttraumatic stress disorder: Evidence for disrupted equilibrium between salience and default mode brain networks. *Psychosomatic Medicine, 74*(9), 904–911.

Staab, J. P., Ruckenstein, M. J., Solomon, D., & Shepard, N. T. (2002). Serotonin reuptake inhibitors for dizziness with psychiatric symptoms. *Archives of Otolaryngology: Head and Neck Surgery, 128*(5), 554–560.

Steil, R., Dyer, A., Priebe, K., Kleindienst, N., & Bohus, M. (2011). Dialectical behavior therapy for posttraumatic stress disorder related to childhood sexual abuse: A pilot study of an intensive residential treatment program. *Journal of Traumatic Stress, 24*(1), 102–106.

Stein, B. E., & Stanford, T. R. (2008). Multisensory integration: Current issues from the perspective of the single neuron. *Nature Reviews: Neuroscience, 9*(4), 255–266.

Stephani, C., Fernandez-Baca Vaca, G., Maciunas, R., Koubeissi, M., & Luders, H. O. (2011). Functional neuroanatomy of the insular lobe. *Brain Structure and Function, 216*(2), 137–149.

Sterling, P. (2012). Allostasis: A model of predictive regulation. *Physiology and Behavior, 106*(1), 5–15.

Steuwe, C., Daniels, J. K., Frewen, P. A., Densmore, M., Pannasch, S., Beblo, T., et al. (2014). Effect of direct eye contact in PTSD related to interpersonal trauma: An fMRI study of activation of an innate alarm system. *Social Cognitive and Affective Neuroscience, 9*(1), 88–97.

Stickgold, R. (2005). Sleep-dependent memory consolidation. *Nature, 437*, 1272–1278.

Stoltz, J. A., Shannon, K., Kerr, T., Zhang, R., Montaner, J. S., & Wood, E. (2007). Associations between childhood maltreatment and sex work in a cohort of drug-using youth. *Social Science and Medicine, 65*(6), 1214–1221.

Svoboda, E., McKinnon, M. C., & Levine, B. (2006). The functional neuroanatomy of autobiographical memory: A meta-analysis. *Neuropsychologia, 44*(12), 2189–2208.

Takahashi, K., Kayama, Y., Lin, J. S., & Sakai, K. (2010). Locus coeruleus neuronal activity during the sleep–waking cycle in mice. *Neuroscience, 169*(3), 1115–1126.

Tecer, A., Tukel, R., Erdamar, B., & Sunay, T. (2004). Audiovestibular functioning in patients with panic disorder. *Journal of Psychosomatic Research, 57*(2), 177–182.

Teicher, M. H., Samson, J. A., Anderson, C. M., & Ohashi, K. (2016). The effects of childhood maltreatment on brain structure, function and connectivity. *Nature Reviews: Neuroscience, 17*(10), 652–666.

Terpou, B. A., Densmore, M., Theberge, J., Thome, J., Frewen, P., McKinnon, M. C., et al. (2019). The threatful self: Midbrain functional connectivity to cortical midline and parietal regions during subliminal trauma-related processing in PTSD. *Chronic Stress, 3*, 2470547019871369.

Terpou, B. A., Harricharan, S., McKinnon, M. C., Frewen, P., Jetly, R., & Lanius, R. A. (2019). The effects of trauma on brain and body: A unifying role for the midbrain periaqueductal gray. *Journal of Neuroscience Research, 97*(9), 1110–1140.

Terpou, B. A., Lloyd, C. S., Densmore, M., McKinnon, M. C., Theberge, J., Neufeld, R. W. J., et al. (2022). Moral wounds run deep: Exaggerated midbrain functional network connectivity across the default mode network in posttraumatic stress disorder. *Journal of Psychiatry and Neuroscience, 47*(1), E56–E66.

Thomaes, K., Dorrepaal, E., Draijer, N., Jansma, E. P., Veltman, D. J., & van Balkom, A.

J. (2014). Can pharmacological and psychological treatment change brain structure and function in PTSD?: A systematic review. *Journal of Psychiatric Research, 50*, 1–15.

Thome, J., Densmore, M., Terpou, B. A., Theberge, J., McKinnon, M. C., & Lanius, R. A. (2022). Contrasting associations between heart rate variability and brainstem–limbic connectivity in posttraumatic stress disorder and its dissociative subtype: A pilot study. *Frontiers in Behavioural Neuroscience, 16*, 862192.

Trevarthen, C., & Aitken, K. J. (2001). Infant intersubjectivity: Research, theory, and clinical applications. *Journal of Child Psychology and Psychiatry, and Allied Disciplines, 42*(1), 3–48.

Tronick, E., & Beeghly, M. (2011). Infants' meaning-making and the development of mental health problems. *American Psychologist, 66*(2), 107–119.

Trousselard, M., Barraud, P. A., Nougier, V., Raphel, C., & Cian, C. (2004). Contribution of tactile and interoceptive cues to the perception of the direction of gravity. *Brain Research: Cognitive Brain Research, 20*(3), 355–362.

Tsakiris, M., Tajadura-Jimenez, A., & Costantini, M. (2011). Just a heartbeat away from one's body: Interoceptive sensitivity predicts malleability of body-representations. *Proceedings: Biological Sciences, 278*(1717), 2470–2476.

Tulving, E., & Thomson, D. M. (1973). Encoding specificity and retrieval processes in episodic memory. *Psychological Review, 80*(5), 352–373.

Tursich, M., Ros, T., Frewen, P. A., Kluetsch, R. C., Calhoun, V. D., & Lanius, R. A. (2015). Distinct intrinsic network connectivity patterns of post-traumatic stress disorder symptom clusters. *Acta Psychiatrica Scandinavica, 132*(1), 29–38.

Uchino, Y., & Kushiro, K. (2011). Differences between otolith- and semicircular canal-activated neural circuitry in the vestibular system. *Neuroscience Research, 71*(4), 315–327.

Uddin, L. Q., Nomi, J. S., Hebert-Seropian, B., Ghaziri, J., & Boucher, O. (2017). Structure and function of the human insula. *Journal of Clinical Neurophysiology, 34*(4), 300–306.

Valenza, G., Ciò, F. D., Toschi, N., & Barbieri, R. (2024). Sympathetic and parasympathetic central autonomic networks. *Imaging Neuroscience, 2*, 1–17.

van der Kolk, B. A. (1989). The compulsion to repeat the trauma: Re-enactment, revictimization, and masochism. *Psychiatric Clinics of North America, 12*(2), 389–411.

van der Kolk, B. A. (2014). *The body keeps the score: Brain, mind, and body in the healing of trauma.* Viking.

van der Kolk, B. A., Brown, P., & van der Hart, O. (1989). Pierre Janet on post-traumatic stress. *Journal of Traumatic Stress, 2*(4), 365–378.

van der Kolk, B. A., & Fisler, R. (1995). Dissociation and the fragmentary nature of traumatic memories: Overview and exploratory study. *Journal of Traumatic Stress, 8*(4), 505–525.

van der Kolk, B. A., & van der Hart, O. (1991). The intrusive past: The flexibility of memory and the engraving of trauma. *American Imago, 48*(4), 425–454.

van Elk, M., & Blanke, O. (2014). Imagined own-body transformations during passive self-motion. *Psychological Research, 78*(1), 18–27.

van IJzendoorn, M. H. (1995). Adult attachment representations, parental responsiveness, and infant attachment: A meta-analysis on the predictive validity of the Adult Attachment Interview. *Psychological Bulletin, 117*(3), 387–403.

Veldhuizen, M. G., Albrecht, J., Zelano, C., Boesveldt, S., Breslin, P., & Lundstrom, J. N. (2011). Identification of human gustatory cortex by activation likelihood estimation. *Human Brain Mapping, 32*(12), 2256–2266.

Venault, P., Rudrauf, D., Lepicard, E. M., Berthoz, A., Jouvent, R., & Chapouthier, G. (2001). Balance control and posture in anxious mice improved by SSRI treatment. *Neuroreport, 12*(14), 3091–3094.

Vermetten, E., & Bremner, J. D. (2003). Olfaction as a traumatic reminder in posttraumatic stress disorder: Case reports and review. *Journal of Clinical Psychiatry, 64*(2), 202–207.

Volchan, E., Rocha-Rego, V., Bastos, A. F., Oliveira, J. M., Franklin, C., Gleiser, S., et al.

(2017). Immobility reactions under threat: A contribution to human defensive cascade and PTSD. *Neuroscience and Biobehavioral Reviews, 76*(Pt. A), 29–38.

Volchan, E., Souza, G. G., Franklin, C. M., Norte, C. E., Rocha-Rego, V., Oliveira, J. M., et al. (2011). Is there tonic immobility in humans?: Biological evidence from victims of traumatic stress. *Biological Psychology, 88*(1), 13–19.

Voss, P., Thomas, M. E., Cisneros-Franco, J. M., & de Villers-Sidani, E. (2017). Dynamic brains and the changing rules of neuroplasticity: Implications for learning and recovery. *Frontiers in Psychology, 8*, 1657.

Vossel, S., Geng, J. J., & Fink, G. R. (2014). Dorsal and ventral attention systems: Distinct neural circuits but collaborative roles. *Neuroscientist, 20*(2), 150–159.

Wallace, M. T., & Stein, B. E. (2007). Early experience determines how the senses will interact. *Journal of Neurophysiology, 97*(1), 921–926.

Warner, E., Finn, H., Westcott, A., Cook, A., & Blaustein, M. E. (2020). *Transforming trauma in children and adolescents: An embodied approach to somatic regulation, trauma processing, and attachment-building.* North Atlantic Books.

Warner, E., Koomar, J., Lary, B., & Cook, A. (2013). Can the body change the score?: Application of sensory modulation principles in the treatment of traumatized adolescents in residential settings. *Journal of Family Violence, 28*(7), 729–738.

Warner, E., Spinazzola, J., Westcott, A., Gunn, C., & Hodgdon, H. (2014). The body can change the score: Empirical support for somatic regulation in the treatment of traumatized adolescents. *Journal of Child and Adolescent Trauma, 7*(4), 237–246.

Weihe, E., Schutz, B., Hartschuh, W., Anlauf, M., Schafer, M. K., & Eiden, L. E. (2005). Coexpression of cholinergic and noradrenergic phenotypes in human and nonhuman autonomic nervous system. *Journal of Comparative Neurology, 492*(3), 370–379.

Wiens, S. (2005). Interoception in emotional experience. *Current Opinion in Neurology, 18*(4), 442–447.

Williams, M. D., & Hollan, J. D. (1981). The process of retrieval from very long-term memory. *Cognitive Science, 5*(2), 87–119.

Wilson, D. A., & Stevenson, R. J. (2003). The fundamental role of memory in olfactory perception. *Trends in Neuroscience, 26*(5), 243–247.

Wilson, M. (2002). Six views of embodied cognition. *Psychonomic Bulletin and Review, 9*(4), 625–636.

Yehuda, R., Engel, S. M., Brand, S. R., Seckl, J., Marcus, S. M., & Berkowitz, G. S. (2005). Transgenerational effects of posttraumatic stress disorder in babies of mothers exposed to the World Trade Center attacks during pregnancy. *Journal of Clinical Endocrinology and Metabolism, 90*(7), 4115–4118.

Yehuda, R., Halligan, S. L., & Grossman, R. (2001). Childhood trauma and risk for PTSD: Relationship to intergenerational effects of trauma, parental PTSD, and cortisol excretion. *Development and Psychopathology, 13*(3), 733–753.

Yehuda, R., Hoge, C. W., McFarlane, A. C., Vermetten, E., Lanius, R. A., Nievergelt, C. M., et al. (2015). Post-traumatic stress disorder. *Nature Reviews: Disease Primers, 1*, 15057.

Yehuda, R., Steiner, A., Kahana, B., Binder-Brynes, K., Southwick, S. M., Zemelman, S., et al. (1997). Alexithymia in Holocaust survivors with and without PTSD. *Journal of Traumatic Stress, 10*(1), 93–100.

Yeo, S. S., Chang, P. H., & Jang, S. H. (2013). The ascending reticular activating system from pontine reticular formation to the thalamus in the human brain. *Frontiers in Human Neuroscience, 7*, 416.

Ying, X., Luo, J., Chiu, C. Y., Wu, Y., Xu, Y., & Fan, J. (2018). Functional dissociation of the posterior and anterior insula in moral disgust. *Frontiers in Psychology, 9*, 860.

Zaccari, B., Sherman, A. D. F., Higgins, M., & Kelly, U. A. (2024). Trauma center trauma-sensitive yoga versus cognitive processing therapy for women veterans with PTSD who experienced military sexual trauma: A feasibility study. *Journal of the American Psychiatric Nurses Association, 30*(2), 343–354.

Zaki, J., Davis, J. I., & Ochsner, K. N. (2012). Overlapping activity in anterior insula during interoception and emotional experience. *NeuroImage, 62*(1), 493–499.

Zanetti, C. A., Powell, B., Cooper, G., & Hoffman, K. (2011). The Circle of Security intervention: Using the therapeutic relationship to ameliorate attachment security in disorganized dyads. In J. Solomon & C. George (Eds.), *Disorganized attachment and caregiving* (pp. 318–342). Guilford Press.

zu Eulenburg, P., Caspers, S., Roski, C., & Eickhoff, S. B. (2012). Meta-analytical definition and functional connectivity of the human vestibular cortex. *NeuroImage, 60*(1), 162–169.

zu Eulenburg, P., Stephan, T., Dieterich, M., & Ruehl, R. M. (2020). The human vestibular cortex. *ScienceOpen Posters.*

Index

Note. f or t following a page number indicates a figure or a table.